AF894258

Foodborne Pathogens - Recent Advances in Control and Detection

Edited by Alexandre Lamas, Carlos Manuel Franco and Patricia Regal

Published in London, United Kingdom

Foodborne Pathogens - Recent Advances in Control and Detection
http://dx.doi.org/10.5772/intechopen.98159
Edited by Alexandre Lamas, Carlos Manuel Franco and Patricia Regal

Contributors
Stephanie A. Smith, Barakatullah Mohammadi, Natasha Gorkina, Rajani Chowdary Akkina, Vijayalakshmi Payala, Sushma Sharoon Maganti, Yiping Chen, Junping Wen, Junpeng Zhao, Chenxi Huang, Ibrahim Musa Musa Moi, Zuhairu Ibrahim, Bashir Mohammed Abubakar, Yahaya Mohammed Katagum, Auwal Abdullahi, Gandi Ajibji Yiga, Badamasi Abdullahi, Ibrahim Mustapha, Jallaba Ali, Hamisu Maimusa, Halima Oge Katagum, Aisha Muhammad Malami, Aminu Mustapha, Zinat Mahmud, Istifanus Ayuba, Elechi Jasper Okoro Godwin Okoro Godwin, Vidhya Chandrasekaran, Adamu Cornelius Smah, Ekoja Omeyi Faith

© The Editor(s) and the Author(s) 2023
The rights of the editor(s) and the author(s) have been asserted in accordance with the Copyright, Designs and Patents Act 1988. All rights to the book as a whole are reserved by INTECHOPEN LIMITED. The book as a whole (compilation) cannot be reproduced, distributed or used for commercial or non-commercial purposes without INTECHOPEN LIMITED's written permission. Enquiries concerning the use of the book should be directed to INTECHOPEN LIMITED rights and permissions department (permissions@intechopen.com).
Violations are liable to prosecution under the governing Copyright Law.

Individual chapters of this publication are distributed under the terms of the Creative Commons Attribution 3.0 Unported License which permits commercial use, distribution and reproduction of the individual chapters, provided the original author(s) and source publication are appropriately acknowledged. If so indicated, certain images may not be included under the Creative Commons license. In such cases users will need to obtain permission from the license holder to reproduce the material. More details and guidelines concerning content reuse and adaptation can be found at http://www.intechopen.com/copyright-policy.html.

Notice
Statements and opinions expressed in the chapters are these of the individual contributors and not necessarily those of the editors or publisher. No responsibility is accepted for the accuracy of information contained in the published chapters. The publisher assumes no responsibility for any damage or injury to persons or property arising out of the use of any materials, instructions, methods or ideas contained in the book.

First published in London, United Kingdom, 2023 by IntechOpen
IntechOpen is the global imprint of INTECHOPEN LIMITED, registered in England and Wales, registration number: 11086078, 5 Princes Gate Court, London, SW7 2QJ, United Kingdom

British Library Cataloguing-in-Publication Data
A catalogue record for this book is available from the British Library

Additional hard and PDF copies can be obtained from orders@intechopen.com

Foodborne Pathogens - Recent Advances in Control and Detection
Edited by Alexandre Lamas, Carlos Manuel Franco and Patricia Regal
p. cm.
Print ISBN 978-1-80355-903-2
Online ISBN 978-1-80355-904-9
eBook (PDF) ISBN 978-1-80355-905-6

We are IntechOpen, the world's leading publisher of Open Access books

Built by scientists, for scientists

6,200+
Open access books available

168,000+
International authors and editors

185M+
Downloads

156
Countries delivered to

Our authors are among the
Top 1%
most cited scientists

12.2%
Contributors from top 500 universities

BOOK CITATION INDEX
CLARIVATE ANALYTICS
INDEXED

WEB OF SCIENCE™

Selection of our books indexed in the Book Citation Index in Web of Science™ Core Collection (BKCI)

Interested in publishing with us?
Contact book.department@intechopen.com

Numbers displayed above are based on latest data collected.
For more information visit www.intechopen.com

Meet the editors

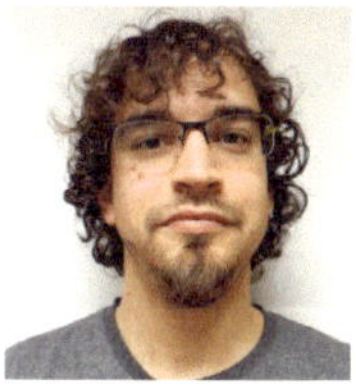

Alexandre Lamas is a full-time assistant professor in the Department of Analytical Chemistry, Nutrition and Bromatology, at the University of Santiago de Compostela, Spain. He obtained a Ph.D. in innovation in food safety technologies from the same university in 2019. He is the author of more than 35 scientific articles in international peer-reviewed journals as well as four book chapters and two chapters in encyclopedias. He is an active reviewer for different food science and microbiology journals and a member of the editorial board of two international journals. His research focuses on the study of foodborne pathogens, especially *Salmonella*, new control methods, the study of food microbiota, and more recently the study of foodborne pathogenic bacteriophages.

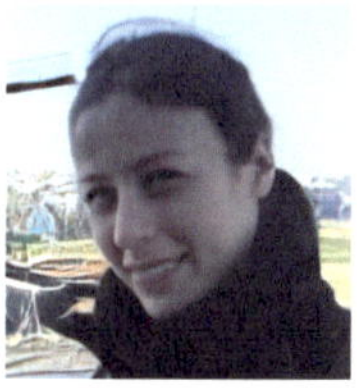

Patricia Regal is a full-time assistant professor in the Department of Analytical Chemistry, Nutrition and Bromatology, at the University of Santiago de Compostela, Spain. She graduated in veterinary science from the Faculty of Veterinary Science of Lugo, in 2007, and obtained her Ph.D. (cum laude) in 2012. Dr. Regal has published more than 50 scientific articles in prestigious international journals. She has co-authored four book chapters, various open-access articles, national contributions, and two chapters in encyclopedias. She has wide practical experience in the fields of food safety, food composition, omic technologies, biostatistics, biomarker discovery, and chromatographic techniques and mass spectrometry applied to biological matrices.

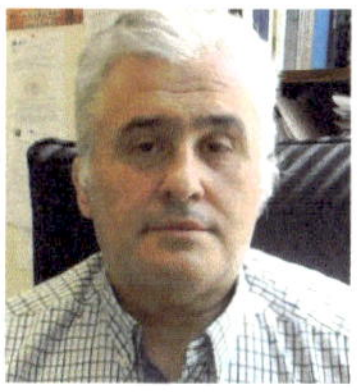

Carlos Manuel Franco is a Full Professor at the University of Santiago de Compostela, in the Department of Analytical Chemistry, Nutrition and Bromatology. He obtained a Ph.D. in nutrition and bromatology from the same university in 1994. He is the author of more than 120 international publications in scientific journals and several book chapters. He is currently a member of the scientific committee of the Spanish Security Agency Food and Nutrition (AESAN). He is the editor-in-chief and an editorial board member of diverse food science and microbiology journals. His research is focused on new methods of food control, the detection of pathogenic bacteria in food and other matrices, and the effect of various substances on pathogenic bacteria.

Contents

Preface IX

Section 1
Foodborne Pathogens: A Global Concern 1

Chapter 1 3
Properties of Foodborne Pathogens and Their Diseases
by Ibrahim Musa Moi, Zuhairu Ibrahim, Bashir Mohammed Abubakar, Yahaya Mohammed Katagum, Auwal Abdullahi, Gandi Ajibji Yiga, Badamasi Abdullahi, Ibrahim Mustapha, Jallaba Ali, Zinat Mahmud, Hamisu Maimusa, Halima Oge Katagum, Aisha Muhammad Malami, Aminu Mustapha and Istifanus Ayuba

Chapter 2 21
Emerging Infectious Food System Related Zoonotic Foodborne Disease – A Threat to Global Food Safety and Nutrition Security
by Elechi Jasper Okoro Godwin, Vidhya Chandrasekaran, Adamu Cornelius Smah and Ekoja Omeyi Faith

Chapter 3 53
Pathogenicity, Toxin Production, Control and Detection of *Bacillus cereus*
by Barakatullah Mohammadi, Natasha Gorkina and Stephanie A. Smith

Section 2
Foodborne Pathogen Dectection Methods 75

Chapter 4 77
Tools for Rapid Detection and Control of Foodborne Microbial Pathogens
by Rajani Chowdary Akkina, Vijayalakshmi Payala and Sharon Sushma Maganti

Chapter 5 97
Advances in the Bacteriophage-Based Precise Identification and Magnetic Relaxation Switch Sensor for Rapid Detection of Foodborne Pathogens
by Yiping Chen, Junping Wen, Junpeng Zhao and Chenxi Huang

Preface

Food safety remains one of the world's major challenges, with foodborne pathogens continuing to cause millions of infections annually worldwide. These infections are of increasing concern due to the rise of antimicrobial-resistant bacteria and so-called super-resistant bacteria. We live in a world where food is distributed globally, so that contamination of food with a pathogenic microorganism in a food factory located in a specific geographic location can cause a worldwide outbreak. One of the measures that has proved most effective globally in preventing foodborne pathogens from reaching the consumer is the establishment of control methods at different points in the food chain. For example, in the European Union, the establishment of national *Salmonella* control plans has resulted in a reduction in the incidence of this pathogen.

In the first chapter, Moi et al. describe the main foodborne pathogens and their diseases. Bacterial pathogens are widely distributed, and disease can be caused by the microorganism itself or by the toxins it produces. Among the main foodborne pathogens, *Campylobacter* spp. and *Salmonella* spp. are responsible for more than 200,000 and 80,000 human cases annually, respectively, in the European Union. Despite the high number of cases, however, the mortality rate is less than 0.2% in the case of *Salmonella* and 0.05% in the case of *Campylobacter*. This contrasts with *Listeria monocytogenes* data showing that although this pathogen is only responsible for about 2,000 reported cases of listeriosis each year in the European Union, it has a mortality rate of 13%. Other types of foodborne pathogens include viruses, parasites and fungi. The latter are of particular concern because of their ability to produce mycotoxins. In Chapter 2, Godwin et al. discuss emerging infectious food system-related zoonotic foodborne disease. Food production needs to increase in line with the increase in the world's population. Food production animals are an important source of foodborne pathogens. Prevention and control measures are therefore essential to avoid increasingly intensive food production resulting in a risk for consumers.

In Chapter 3, Mohammadi and Smith review *Bacillus cereus*. This is a ubiquitous microorganism causing great concern in the food industry due to its ability to survive in a wide range of environmental conditions as well as its capacity to withstand stressful conditions. Toxins produced by this bacterium are responsible for two types of intoxication in humans, diarrheal syndrome and emetic syndrome. The number of cases of food poisoning caused by this foodborne pathogen is underestimated, because it usually produces mild and transient symptoms. However, it is estimated that it is responsible for a high number of annual poisonings worldwide, making its control and detection essential. Detection methods preventing the transmission of pathogens through the food production chain are critical. In Chapter 4, Akkina et al. describe different tools for rapid detection of these problematic microorganisms. In the case of bacteria, classical microbiology methods have always been one of the main reference methods due to their robustness and extensive validation. However, these methods are limited by the time required to obtain the final result, which in some cases, such as *Salmonella*, can take up to a week. In recent years alternative methods have emerged that obtain results more quickly, and methods based on the amplification of nucleic acids have been gaining in importance. For example, real-time PCR is proving to be a valuable tool to accelerate the detection of foodborne pathogens, alone or in combination with classical microbiology methods. Similarly, in recent years there has been a growing interest in biosensors. In Chapter 5, Chen et al. discuss the use of bacteriophages (phages) as a valuable tool to detect foodborne pathogens. Phages are viruses that infect only bacteria and are characterized by their specificity, each phage normally only infecting a specific species of bacteria or even only some strains. Part of the phage's surface binds specifically to some bacterial surface molecules, which are responsible for their range of activity. Both whole phages and some of their parts can be used to detect pathogens, so these viruses have great potential in the design of new diagnostic tools.

We are enormously grateful to all the authors who have contributed to making this book a reality. We are also very grateful to the entire Intech team for their invaluable help throughout the process of preparing this book, and especially to Zrinka Tomicic, whose help has been essential to enabling this book to go ahead.

Alexandre Lamas, Carlos Manuel Franco and Patricia Regal
LHICA,
Department of Analytical Chemistry,
Nutrition and Bromatology,
Universidade de Santiago de Compostela,
Lugo, Spain

Section 1

Foodborne Pathogens: A Global Concern

Chapter 1

Properties of Foodborne Pathogens and Their Diseases

Ibrahim Musa Moi, Zuhairu Ibrahim, Bashir Mohammed Abubakar, Yahaya Mohammed Katagum, Auwal Abdullahi, Gandi Ajibji Yiga, Badamasi Abdullahi, Ibrahim Mustapha, Jallaba Ali, Zinat Mahmud, Hamisu Maimusa, Halima Oge Katagum, Aisha Muhammad Malami, Aminu Mustapha and Istifanus Ayuba

Abstract

Thousands of foodborne pathogens are causing a great number of diseases with significant effects on human health and economy. Foodborne pathogens can contaminate food items not only during production and processing, but also at the time of storage and transport before consuming. During their growth, these microorganisms are capable of secreting different type of toxins into the extracellular environment. Likewise, other harmful substances can be also released and can contaminate food after breakup of food pathogens. Many microbial toxins can withstand inactivation, and can endure harsh treatment during food processing. Many of these molecules are partaken in cellular processes and can display different mechanisms of pathogenesis of foodborne organisms. Thus studying the properties of foodborne pathogens can help in the understanding of their contamination and inactivation. In the present review, we discussed extensively on the properties of foodborne pathogens including bacteria, viruses and parasites. In addition, some of the diseases caused by foodborne pathogens and the mechanism of their pathogenesis were also discussed.

Keywords: properties, foodborne disease, viruses, bacteria, fungi

1. Introduction

Pathogenic microorganisms such as bacteria, virus, fungi and parasite caused foodborne diseases, however, bacteria are the most common cause of foodborne pathogen and exist in a variety of shapes, types and properties. Some are capable of spore formation and thus, highly heat-resistant (e.g. *Clostridium botulinum, Clostridium perfringens, Bacillus subtilus, Bacillus cereus*). Some are capable of producing heat-resistant toxins (e.g. *Staphylococcus aureus, C. botulinum*). Most are mesophilic with optimal growth temperature range from 20–45°C. Moreover, certain foodborne pathogens (i.e. psychrotrophs), such as *Listeria monocytogenes*, and *Yersinia enterocolitica* are capable of growing under refrigerated conditions or temperatures less than 10°C. Common disease associated with foodborne pathogens include botulism, cholera, typhoid, dysentery, listeriosis and many more. Foodborne illness is typically caused by micro-organisms or their toxins and most often manifests itself through gastrointestinal illness, which can vary markedly in severity and duration [1]. The zoonotic characteristics of foodborne pathogens and their capability to generate toxins causing diseases or even death are enough to consider the genuineness of the circumstances. Foodborne pathogens cause tremendous of cases of sporadic infections and chronic difficulties, as well as huge and terrible outbreaks in several countries and between countries. The degree of this problem is confirmed by the considerable number of the 1.5 billion annual diarrheal cases in children below 3 years of age that are caused by enteropathogenic microorganisms, which leads to more than 3 million deaths per year [2]. Report has indicated that in the United States alone, bacterial enteric pathogens cause 9.4 million cases of foodborne infection in humans, 55,961 hospitalizations, and 1,351 deaths each year [2]. The rapid increase of residents and urbanization, the level income per capita, the industrialization, the changes of the purchaser habits (eating more protein in the diet) have escalated the consumption of animal products [3]. Analysis proposed that consumption of these products will get higher to 376 million tons by 2030 [3]. This huge demand of animal products has triggered animal production and processing of products, with an increase of foods transportation worldwide. This condition could lead to substandard processing practices and enhance of the risk of contamination by foodborne pathogens at any place. Animal and animal products contamination is a major public health concern because it is hard to manage. Several factors could cause this contamination including water from different sources, frequent disposal of animal's manure, and improper handling of animal during slaughtering and processing practices, and storage procedures [2]. Foodborne pathogens are capable of causing disease through consumption of the animal products polluted with microorganisms or their toxins. This chapter reviewed the properties and diseases of foodborne pathogens comprising bacteria, fungi viruses, and parasites. In addition, the mechanism through which these foodborne pathogens caused disease has also reviewed.

2. Common foodborne pathogens and their properties

2.1 Bacterial pathogens

Bacteria are the most widely foodborne pathogens causing numerous foodborne diseases either by ingestion of the microorganisms themselves or toxins produced by certain groups microorganisms. Common bacteria found in foods include but not limited to the following: V. *cholera*, *C. botulinum*, *C. perfringens*, *E. coli*, *S. aureus*, *Salmonella* species, *Shigella* species, *Listeria monocytogens*, Bacillus species, Yersinia species, Campylobacter species. They range from Gram-positive, Gram-negative, cocci to bacillus or rod shape. Some are aerobic, while others are anaerobic, some are psychrophiles, mesophiles while others are thermophiles, some bacteria form spores while others are non-spore forming. These foodborne bacteria are discussed in detail below.

2.1.1 Vibrio cholerae

V. cholerae is a Gram negative rod (comma) or curved shaped facultative anaerobe bacterium that ranges from 0.7–1.0 by 1.5–3.0 μm in size. It thrives well on thiosulfate citrate bile salts sucrose (TCBS) agar, upon growing on TCBS, the pathogen produces pale-yellow, shining (translucent) colonies 3 mm in diameter *V. cholerae*is one of the most abundant species of Vibros that causes infections to humans apart from *Vibrio parahaemolyticus* and *Vibrio vulnificus.* The pathogen undergoes two (2) lifestyles; as a free-living when it inside aquatic environment or pathogenic when in the gastrointestinal tract. It has the ability to remain virulent without multiplying in fresh water and sea water for a long time. They are numerous in temperate waters and can be isolated in seafood and fish. The most notable species are *V. cholerae*O1 and O139, causative serogroups of cholera. Non-O1 strains and the rest of about 9 species cause cholera-like diarrheal syndromes, but they are not as severe, even though they frequently produce extra intestinal infections. The CTX toxin (Cholera toxin) is the main virulence factor of *V. cholerae*O1 [4]. *V. cholerae* has a single polar flagellum located at the extreme side of the bacterium which enables it to move (motility) from one place to another and colonization across the intestinal mucosa. However, there are other virulent factors that helps the organism survive or damage the host cell, these include; lipopolysaccharide (LPS), biotin, flagellin, iron-regulated outer membrane proteins [5].

2.1.2 C. perfringens

C. perfringens is a Gram-positive, spore forming, anaerobic bacillus about 3.0–8.0 by 0.4–1.2 μm in size. They are mesophiles that is they can grow well at some moderate temperatures between 20–45°C. C perfringens is a fastidious non-motile bacterium that shows hemolysis when growing on blood agar. Because they are too demanding and requires much vitamins and amino acids for growth and multiplication, hence, they thrive well in meat products because meat product contains high amount of vitamins and amino acids especially beef meat [6]. It's virulence factors are incorporated within the plasmids, these include but not limited to alpha toxin (phospholipase C), kappa toxin (Collagenase), beta epsilon, iota toxins, delta toxins (hemolysins), theta toxins (streptolysin O) [7].

2.1.3 C. botulinum

C. botulinum are Gram-positive, catalase negative, motile, spore-forming, obligate anaerobic rod bacterium about 4.0–6.0 μm in size. They are Psychrophiles which grow at a temperature ranges between 3 and 15°C, however, proteolytic strains thrive well at an optimum temperature of 35–37°C, however, non-proteolytic strains grow well at a temperature ranges between 26 and 28°C respectively. Its virulent factors include toxin: botulinum neurotoxin (BoNT) which specifically damage the neurons, C2 and C3 toxins which causes cell damage and helps in spreading botulinum toxin in the tissue, flagella [8]. *C. botulinum* are motile by means of peritrichous flagella. There are seven types of botulinum neurotoxin; A through G, based on the antigenic specificity of the toxin produced by each strain [9].

2.1.4 L. monocytogenes

L. monocytogenes are Gram-positive rods, non-spore forming bacterium that contained peritrichous flagellation with tumbling motility. They range from 1 to 2 μm in size, which exist as either single or double cells. They are psychrophiles which grow well at a temperature range from 1 to 45°C [10]. The organism is cultured under aerobic conditions on blood agar which formed small gray colonies surrounded by discreet hemolytic zone, caused by listeriolysin O. [11]. They occur ubiquitously in nature and they are present in many food products, mainly in soft cheeses, dairy products, and many cheeses made with unpasteurized milk, celery, cabbage, ice cream, hot dogs, and processed meats [12].

2.1.5 B. cereus

B. cereus are Gram-positive, motile rods, spore-forming bacterium which is about 0.5 × 1.2–2.5 × 10 μm in diameter in size. Most Bacillus spp. Are predominantly found as free-living in nature, they are present in soils, fresh and marine water environments. *B. cereus* produced spores which are hydrophobic in nature with many attachments (appendages) and/or pili. The spores are the virulent factor of *B. cereus* which enable the bacterium to adsorbed firmly to different types of surfaces and do repel removal during disinfection. Vegetative cells of *B. cereus* grow at temperatures ranging from 4 to 15 to 35–55°C [13].

2.1.6 Campylobacter jejuni

*C. jejuni*are members of the family Campylobacteriaceae and is one of the most common cause of diarrheal illness. *C. jejuni*is responsible for approximately 850,000 illnesses, 8,500 hospitalizations, and 76 deaths in the US each year. Based on staining characteristics, the pathogen is biochemically, *C. jejuni*is a Gram- negative consisting of thin layer of peptidoglycan in their cell wall, catalase positive, oxidase positive, urease negative. Morphologically, they exist in spiral or helical rods (S-shape), they do not form spore (non-spore-forming organism) and occur mostly from 0.5–5.0 μm in length. *C. jejuni*possessed a polar flagellation with one at both end and undergoes twisting-like locomotion. Culturally, C. *jejuni*is a fastidious and most successful foodborne microbe that has a rigorous growth conditions, in terms of oxygen concentration, *C. jejuni* is microaerophilic organism which require oxygen concentration as low as 3–5% and carbon dioxide concentration range from 3 to 10% respectively. Unlike other gram negative organism, *C. jejuni* are thermophiles that grow well at 42°C, they consume amino acids instead of carbohydrates for growth, hence, require complex media for growth artificially [14].

2.1.7 Escherichia coli

E. coli is a Gram-negative, catalase positive, oxidase negative, VP negative, indole positive, urease and citrate negative, non-spore forming rod about 1.0–2.0 μm in size. Some are motile with the means of flagella while others are non-motile. They are facultative anaerobe, because they utilize carbohydrate during growth on artificial media, hence, they convert glucose to lactic, acetic, and formic acids as byproducts; however, in terms pH concentrations, *E. coli* grow at an optimum pH of 6.0 to 8.0 (i.e., they grow well in alkaline as well as in acidic environment). *E. coli* comprise a large and diverse group of bacteria with majority harmless strains; other strains are pathogenic and are harmful, thus, have acquired characteristics, such toxins production, which make them pathogenic to humans [15]. Based on the pathogenicity and mechanism of pathogenicity, *E. coli* have been categorized into six groups: (1) Enteropathogenic*E. coli* (EPEC); (2) Enterohemorrhagic*E. coli* (EHEC, also known as Shiga toxin-producing *E. coli* [STEC] and formerly referred to as verotoxin-producing *E. coli* [VTEC]);

(3) Enterotoxigenic*E. coli* (ETEC); (4) Enteroaggregative*E. coli* (EAggEC); (5) Enteroinvasive*E. coli* (EIEC) are non-motile, lactose negative, lysin dicarboxylic negative. EIEC are biochemically, genetically and pathogenetically associated to *Shigellaspp*, like *Shigella*spp, EIEC causes watery diarrhea and dysentry; and (6) Attaching and Effacing *E. coli* (A/EEC) also known diffusely adhering *E. coli* (DAEC) [16].

2.1.8 S. aureus

S. aureus are Gram-positive cocci bacterium which exists as single (monococcus), pairs as in (diplococci), tetrads or short chains (Streptococci) or grape-like clusters (Staphylococci) and gliacoccus based on cellular arrangements. *S. aureus* is one of the abundant normal flora of animals including humans which are predominantly found on the skin, blood, mammary glands, intestine, genitals, respiratory tracts and mouth. They are non-motile, non-spore forming bacterium of about. 0.5–1.5 μm in size which are able to proliferate rapidly in aerobic environments [9]. Under normal condition, and when grown in immunocompetent individual *S. aureus* is non-pathogenic and form a communalistic relationship (Commensalism), however, when they change environment apart from where they are naturally found or when the host immunity is weakened or become compromised, they become opportunistic and caused what is called opportunistic infections (OIs). *S. aureus* can remain dormant outside human body for a long period of time in air, sewage, water and dust, apart from environmental sources, *S. aureus* can be found in foods such as beef, turkey, pork sausage, oysters, milk, salads, cream pies. Depending on the strain, *S. aureus* grow at a temperatures ranging from 7 to 48C [9]. Biochemically, *S. aureus* is catalase positive, coagulase positive and ferment mannitol. *S. aureus* produces a family of virulence factors such as adhesion proteins such as fibronectin, fibrinogen, teichoic acid, enolase, biofilm-associated proteins, enterotoxins such as staphylococcal enterotoxins, super antigens such as Toxic Shock Syndrome Toxin (TST), exfoliative toxins (A, B), hemolysins such as alpha, beta, gamma and delta hemolysins, ADP-ribosylating toxins such as leucocidin, pyrogenic exotoxin, and enzymes (proteases) such as collagenase, Hyaluronidase, Endopeptidase, Elastase [17].

2.1.9 Salmonella spp.

The genus Salmonella belongs to the family Enterobacteriaciae mostly coliform which are indicators. The present of such organisms in water indicated that the water is contaminated with fecal material. Morphologically, Salmonella possess peritrichous flagella which enable the organism to locomote or move from one place to another in the living host, they are non-spore-forming, Gram-negative rods bacterium [18]. These Salmonella were named after the scientist Dr. Daniel Salmon who isolated the first organism, *Salmonella choleraesuis*, from the intestine of a pig. The genus *Salmonella* is divided into two species that can cause illness in humans: *Salmonella enterica and Salmonella bongori*. *Salmonella* is further subdivided into serotypes, based on the Kaufmann-White typing scheme first published in 1934, which differentiates *Salmonella* strains by their surface and flagellar antigenic properties [19].

2.1.10 Shigella spp.

The genus *Shigella*is a member of the family E*nterobacteriaceae*and possesses four serogroupsthat have been traditionally treated as species: serogroup A as

Shigelladysenteriae, serogroup B as *Shigellaflexneri,* serogroup C as *Shigellaboydii,* and, serogroup D as *Shigellasonnei.* Whereas serogroups A, B, and C consist of 38 serotypes, serogroup D possesses only one [20]. They are Gram-negative, non-motile, non-spore forming rod and facultative anaerobic bacterium. Based on staining and biochemical characteristics, Shigellaspp are catalase-positive, but oxidase and lactose negative respectively. They are good fermenters of sugars and grow well at an optimum temperature 37°C, however, other strains grow at less or greater temperature. Their virulence factors are encoded within their extra chromosomal material called plasmid [21]. Plasmid is located in the chromosome of the bacterium; it contains genes that aid the organism during reproduction.

2.1.11 Y. enterocolitica

The genus *Yersinia* belongs to the family *Enterobacteriaceae*and includes ten (10) established species. They are Gram-negative usually short rod bacterium; non-spore-forming, facultative anaerobes which grow at the temperature ranges between 0 and 44°C however, require optimum temperature range between 24.5–28.5°C. Some species are motile with the aid of flagella while others are non-flagellated, hence, they are non-motile. The swimming and/or swarming motility is dependent upon the temperature of the surrounding environment. At 25°C the organism is able to grow peritrichous flagella, while at 37°C, they are non-motile because they do not possess flagella. Based on cultural characteristics, *Y. enterocolitica*grows slowly on MacConkey agar, blood agar, they are good fermenters of sugars (sucrose) but not lactose or xylose. Yersinia can grow in both environment/food and in human bodies, thus, they undergo two types of lifecycles (diphasic). *Yersinia pestis*is the causative agent of plague, *Yersinia pseudotuberculosis* is primarily an animal pathogen but may infect humans after the ingestion of contaminated food or water, and *Y. enterocolitica* has surfaced as a cause of foodborne gastroenteritis in humans [22]. Based on the degree of infectivity, ecologic and geographic distributions, *Y. enterocolitica*are classified into five (5) groups and 60 serotypes namely: 1(A and B), 2, 3, 4 and 5 respectively. It is not all Yersinia strains that are virulent, some virulent Yersinia stains have their virulent factors encoded within their plasmid, these virulence plasmids are called pVY. They aid in adhesion, invasion and colonization of intestinal epithelial cells and lymph nodes [23].

2.2 Viral pathogen

Viruses are inert, obligate ultramicroscopic parasites. They possess either RNA or DNA but not both. They may be enveloped or non-envelope, symmetrical or asymmetrical, segmented or unsegmented, helical, or icosahedral in shape. Unlike bacteria, and other microorganisms, virus are non-cellular and as such they cannot be cultured on artificial culture media. Some viruses that causes foodborne are discuss in details below.

2.2.1 Hepatitis a virus *(HAV)*

Hepatitis A virus particle belong to the family Picornaviridae and genus Heparnavirus also called enterovirus 72. This pathogen, genetically, it is a non-enveloped single stranded positive sense polarity RNA, icosahedral virus with about 7.5 kb and 27 nm in diameter in size. Despite genetic heterogeneity, HAV has only one serotype group but multiple genotypes. However, genotypes I and III are most prevalent affecting humans. Because of it morphological characteristics, HAV can remain viable on the environmental surfaces for a long period of time under favorable environmental conditions such as temperature, pressure and humidity. However, when on human hands, it can remain viable for many hours to few days. HAV can also remain viable in sewage and water bodies for several weeks despite freezing. Serologically, the present of immunoglobulin M (IgM) is indicative of the virus hepatitis A [24]. Recently, outbreaks of viral gastroenteritis and Hepatitis A have been associated with eating usually uncooked shellfish. A clam-associated outbreak of Hepatitis A in Shanghai may have been the largest recorded outbreak of foodborne disease in history, with 292,301 cases [25].

2.2.2 Noroviruses

Norovirus is a non-enveloped single-stranded positive sense RNA which belongs to the family Caliciviridae, genus Lagovirus, or Vesivirus [26]. Most Novoviruses are classified into five (5) genogroups, and in some textbooks six (6) from GI-VI, however, most human infections resulting from genogroups GI and GII. The genome is about 7.5 kb in length and encodes for about three open reading frames (ORFs): ORF1,2 and 3. ORF1 encodes a large polyprotein that is post-translationally cleaved into six nonstructural proteins which include the RNA-dependent RNA polymerase (RdRp), while ORF2 and ORF3 codes for major (Viral protein, VP1) and minor (VP2) capsid proteins respectively [27]. Majority of acute viral gastroenteritis cases worldwide, including an estimated 5.4 million episodes of foodborne illnesses in the US annually are usually caused by norovirus, it is also the leading cause of pediatric acute gastroenteritis particularly among children under the age of 5 [28]. The virus's abilities to withstand a wide range of temperatures (from freezing to 60°C) and to persist on environmental surfaces and food items contribute to rapid dissemination, particularly via secondary spread (via food handlers or to family members) [29].

2.2.3 Bird-flu virus

Bird-Flu Virus also called avian influenza virus or influenza virus belongs to family Orthomyxoviridae, genus influenza virus. The virus is classified into three: Influenza virus A, B and C, however, type A influenza virus is the most important of the three types. Because of the changes or alterations in antigenic structure due to point mutation within narrower range and recombination within broader range which occur less frequently than the latter, influenza type A virus is the major pathogen responsible for epidemics and pandemics. However, type B tends to be endemics more than type C. influenza virus is the pathogen responsible for flu, whereby, the clinical picture or manifestations is associated with bacterial co-infection such as pneumonia. Genetically, influenza virus contains single-stranded RNA, while morphologically, it is segmented, nucleocapsid, and spike proteins which are encapsulated within a structure called envelope. It also contains other proteins such as hemagglutinin, neuraminidase which help in viral pathogenicity and pathogenesis. As earlier said, the genome of influenza virus has about eight separate antisense RNA strands and mostly segmented which encodes for separate and specific proteins each [11].

2.3 Parasites

Parasites are eukaryotic protozoans which exists in various shapes and forms. They have true nucleus which is enclosed within a nuclear membrane.

Some parasites have mitochondria while absent in others. Others organelles present in their cytoplasm include but not limited to endoplasmic reticulum, ribosomes, flagella, pseudopods, cilia. Parasitic organisms that causes foodborne illness are discussed below.

2.3.1 Toxoplasma gondii

*Toxoplasma gondii*is an obligate intracellular microscopic protozoan which belong to the phylum *Apicomplexa*, itcauses toxoplasmosis in humans. Its life cycle consists of two phases: intestinal (enteroepithelial) phase and extra intestinal phase. The intestinal phase is taking place mostly in the primary host such as cats; while the extra intestinal phase is mostly seen in all animals including humans. However, humans and other mammals are the intermediate hosts. The pathogen has three (3) stages in its lifecycle; Tachyzoites, bradyzoites and sporozoites, however, tachyzoites (endozoites) and bradyzoites (cystozoites) takes place in the tissues, whereas tachyzoites multiply and damage infected host cells by means endodyogeny (the formation of two daughter cells from mother cells by means of budding, while the bradyzoites proliferate inside the tissue cysts [4].

2.3.2 Giadia lamblia

*Giardia duodenalis*also known as *Giardia lamblia* or *Gasterophilus intestinalis* is responsible for giardiasis. The pathogen consists of two stages oflife cycle: trophozoite (a jewel shape, non-infective stage, about 9–21 m long and 5–15 μm wide, and contain nuclei with four flagella) and cyst (ovoid; 9–12 m long, resistant and highly infective and matured stage). Infective dose is 10–100 cysts and the incubation period is 1–2 weeks. Reproduction is by asexual means through binary fission. Because it is flagellated organism, G*iadialimblia*undergoes tumbling motility [4].

2.3.3 Entamoeba histolytica

*E. histolytica*is a pathogenic and the most invasive member of the genus and is responsible for amebic dysentery. It exists in two forms morphologically, as a cyst and as a trophozoite. The cyst of *E. coli* is about 0–15 μm in diameter, and are highly infective in nature, while the trophozoites are usually 10–60 μmin diameter, non-motile and do adhere and invade intestinal epithelial cells. Their virulence factors include Gal/GalNAc-inhibitable lectin which a pivotal role in adhesion and tissue demolition, these virulence factors also help the pathogen to interact with host glycoprotein to adhere (adsorb), to block complement activation, as well as to promote cytotoxicity of neutrophils and macrophages. *E. coli* also produced a structure called amoebapore which cannels ions in to the host cell membrane causing cytolysis. The genus *Entamoeba* comprises of a number of species: *E. histolytica, E. dispar, E. moshkovski, E. coli, Entamoeba hartmanni*, and *Entamoeba polecki*. Others exist as commensals in human intestine. E. *histolytica*produces amoebapore that forms ion channels in the host cell membrane causing cytolysis. Each trophozoite carries single nucleus and can convert into precyst and matures into tetra nucleated cysts which are released with feces. Cysts can survive outside the body for several weeks to months if the temperature is favorable (−5°C or over 40°C) [4].

2.3.4 Ascaris lumbricoids

Ascarislumbricoids, A nematode that parasitize in the small intestine of humans, The adult worm (giant round worm) is about 15–40 cm in length, yellowish pin in color and thick as pencil. The sexually matured female Ascaris produce about 200 000 eggs per day usually in unembrayonated state which are then released in feces. The eggs of A. *limbricoides* which exist in spherical or oval in shape are about 60 x 45 um in size, with thick brownish shell and uneven shape. It takes almost three to 6 weeks for an egg to develop into larval stage at optimum temperature from 20–25°C, sufficient water (moisture) and oxygen [11]. They are associated with food when prepared under poor sanitary conditions [4].

2.4 Fungal pathogens

Fungal are eukaryotic organisms unlike bacteria which are prokaryotic. Depending on the temperature upon which the fungal cells are growing, fungal pathogens exists in two forms: (as a molds, and as a yeasts). The phenomenon of which they are grown is called dimorphism. Dimorphism is the phenomenon whereby fungal cells exists in two forms based on the temperature, at $2^{0}5$ C, the fungi exists as molds e.g.; *Aspergillus* species, while at 37°C they exist as a yeast e.g. *Candida albicans*. Unlike bacteria in which their cell wall consist of peptidoglycan, fungal cell wall constitute primarily of chitin (which is a polysaccharide composed of long chains of N-acetylglucoseamine). They reproduced both sexually and asexually, some fungal hyphae are segmented hence, they are called septate while others are unsegmented, thus, they are aseptate. Most fungal cell walls consist of ergosterol. Details explanation on fungal pathogens that are associated with foodborne diseases are discussed below.

2.4.1 Aspergillus flavus

A.*flavus*are multicellular microorganisms and a typical mold possesses hyphae, conidiophore—consisting of stalk, vesicle, sterigmata, and conidia. They produced mycotoxin called Aflatoxin, which exist in different chemical forms; B1, B2, G1, G2, and M1. The B and G stand for blue fluorescence and green fluorescence, respectively. Aflatoxins are found in nuts, spices, and figs and produced during storage under hot and humid conditions. The allowable toxin limits are 20 ppb in nuts (example, Brazilnuts, peanuts, pistachio). Aflatoxin contaminated feed causes high mortality in farm animals. These aflatoxins cause harm in human body in three ways: mutagenic- they caused mutation either in the form of substitution, frame-shift, deletion and/or addition mutation which cause infection of the liver (hepatotoxic), Teratogenic action leads to birth defects and the carcinogenic effect cause irreversible defects in cell physiology resulting in abnormal cell growth and metastasis (called cancer or tumor) [4].

2.4.2 Aspergillus ochraceus

These are microscopic molds fungi consist of hyphae, conidiophore and conidia. They produced mycotoxin called ochratoxin. It is found in a large variety of foods including wheat, corn, soybeans, oats, barley, coffee beans, meats and cheese however, barley is thought to be the predominant source. Ochratoxin is hepatotoxic and nephrotoxic and a potent teratogen and carcinogen. Nephropathy and renal problem are predominant consequences of ochratoxin poisoning. It inhibits cellular function by inhibiting the synthesis of phenylalanine–tRNA complex, and ATP production. It also stimulates lipid peroxidation. The LD50 value in rats is between 20 and 22 mg kg^{-1} [30].

2.4.3 Fussarium spp

These microscopic saprophytic, filamentous fungi that belong to the hyphomycetes. The genus Fussarium has over 300species. They reproduce asexually by spore production. Fusarium species produced three kinds of asexual spores; microconidia, macroconidia and chlamydospores respectively. However, the spore formation defends on the type of specie, some species produces three while others produce only one. Microconidia are developed in conidiophores, these microconidia are produced in the aerial mycelium with different shapes and sizes. They caused variety of plant and animal disease including humans. Their ability to cause disease is based on the ability to produce mycotoxins. Some mycotoxins produced by some species of Fussarium include; fumonosins, zearalenone (F*ussariumgraminearum*). Fumonosins are water soluble compound which are produced by the condensation of amino acid alanine into acetate. It is abundant as fumonosin B1. They cause variety of disease in humans such as leukoencephalomalacia, pulmonary edema, hydrothorax and esophageal cancers [4]. Zearalenone is a mycoestrogen produced by F*ussariumgraminearum*in the human ovary which result to infertility in humans [30].

2.4.4 Penicilliumpatulum

Penicillium is a saprophytic microscopic fungus, commonly known as blue or green mold. Their vegetative thallus or body called mycelium is copiously branched with septate (cross-wall) hyphae range from unicellular to multicellular in nature that reproduces by sexual, asexual and vegetative means. They produced a conidiospores during asexual reproduction which are non-motile and are developed inside a conidiophore as well as an ascospores. They produced secondary metabolites called patulin. Bread, sausage, fruits (apricots, grapes, peaches, pears, and apples), and apple juice are the major source of this toxin. Patulin is a carcinogen and is reported to be responsible for subcutaneous sarcoma, it must be present in high quantity for as much as 15–25 mg kg – 1 (LD50 value) for infection to occur [30].

2.4.5 Penicilliumcitrinum

P*enicilliumcitrinum*is a saprophytic microscopic fungus, commonly known as blue or green mold. Their vegetative thallus or body called mycelium is copiously branched with septate (cross-wall) hyphae range from unicellular to multicellular in nature that reproduces by sexual, asexual and vegetative means. They produced a conidiospores during asexual reproduction which are non-motile and are developed inside a conidiophore as well as an ascospores. These fungal pathogens produced a mycotoxin called citrinin. The major source of this toxin is rice, moldy bread, ham, wheat, oats, rye and barley. Citrinin is a nephrotoxin and causes nephropathy in animals. It is reported that the LD50 value for citrinin in chicken is 95 mg kg – 1; in rabbits, 134 mg kg – 1 and its significance in human health is unknown [4].

DOI: http://dx.doi.org/10.5772/intechopen.105694

2.4.6 Clavicepspurpurea

Clavicepspurpurea is some microscopic saprophytic fungi with septate hyphae. It *produces* a toxic cocktail of alkaloid, which is not considered a typical mycotoxin. Ergots grow on the heads of grasses such as wheat and ryes and the disease is known as St Anthony's Fire because of severe burning sensations in the limbs and extremities of the victim. Two forms of egotism are reported: gangrenous and convulsive. In the gangrenous form, the blood supply is affected causing tissue damage. In the convulsive form, the toxin affects the central nervous system. The egotism is a serious problem in animals including cattle, sheep, pigs and chicken resulting in gangrene, convulsions, abortion, hypersensitivity and ataxia. In cattle, ergotism spreads around the hooves and animal may lose hooves and are unable to walk and die by starvation [30]

3. Common disease associated with food

The **Table 1** describes some common foodborne diseases caused by bacteria, viruses, parasites and fungal pathogens respectively including the mode of transmission/food associated and clinical manifestation.

Diseases	Pathogen	Mode of transmission and associated food	Clinical Manifestations	Reference
Cholera	*Vibrocholerae*	Fecal-oral route via vegetables, seafood, rice and beans	Vomiting, watery diarrhea, dehydration, loss of appetite, fever, weakness of the body, headache, malaise.	[31]
Enteritis	*Clostridium perfringens*	Ingestion of beef and poultry meat	Vomiting, abdominal pains, fever, dizziness, putrefactive diarrhea.	[32]
Botulism	*Clostridium botulinum*	Ingestion of toxin-preformed food such as vegetables, pepper, meat, fish and baked potatoes	Diarrhea, fever, vomiting, eyes disturbance, weakness of the muscles, dizziness, constipation, fatigue, dry mouth, respiratory track failure, heart attack, paralysis, vertigo.	[33]
Listeriosis	*Listeria monocytogens*	Ingestion of food such as raw milk, soft cheese, meat based paste, jellied pork tongue, raw vegetables and coleslaw	Gastrointestinal discomfort, fever, headache, athalgia, malady, chills, swollen nymph nodes.	[34]
Gastroenteritis	*Bacillus cereus*	Ingestion of contaminated food such raw milk and raw or undercooked poultry is the mode of transmission	Diarrhea, nausea, abdominal pain, vomiting.	[35]
Escherichia coli infection	*E. coli*	Consumption of food and water contaminated with fecal matter. Food involved include; vegetables, raw milk, ground meat,	Vomiting, diarrhea (bloody, mucus), nausea, fever, abdominal cramps.	[36]

Diseases	Pathogen	Mode of transmission and associated food	Clinical Manifestations	Reference
Intoxication	*Staphylococcus aureus*	Consumption of foods containing the toxin. Example of food include meat, rice, raw milk, stew.	Nausea, vomiting, diarrhea, adoration (prostration), constipation, heaving, abdominal discomfort.	[9]
Typhoid and paratyphoid fever	*Salmonella typhi*and *paratyphi*	Transmission is via ingestion of food and water contaminated with fecal matter such as raw milk, meat, selfish, salad.	Excessive fever, vomiting, headache, abdominal pains, constipation, diarrhea, psychosis in some cases, chills, rose spot, cough.	[37]
Yersiniosis	*Yersinia enterocolitica.*	is transmitted through consumption of pork products (tongue, tonsils, gut), cured or uncured, as well as milk and milk products	Diarrhea, vomiting, fever, abdominal cramp.	[22]
Shigellosis (bacillary dysentery)	*Shigelladysentriae*	Ingestion of food and water contaminated with fecal matter such as salads and vegetables; water, raw milk	Diarrhea containing blood, pus and mucus, abdominal discomfort, fever, vomiting.	[38]
Hepatitis A	Hepatitis A Virus	Transmitted fecal-orally in food and drinking water such as shellfish, raw fruit and vegetables, bakery products	Nausea, loss of appetite, fever, vomiting, inflammation of the liver, jaundice, dark urine.	[39]
Viral gastroenteritis	Norovirus(Norwalk virus)	Fecal-orally in drinking water and food. E.g. shellfish or drinking water contaminated with sewage	Diarrhea, fever, vomiting, abdominal pain, dehydration.	[39]
Bird flu or avian influenza	Bird flu virus or influenza virus or avian influenza virus	Fecal-orally in food and drinking water	Fever, headache, coughing, flu, vomiting, diarrhea.	[11]
Viral gastroenteritis	Rotavirus or Adenovirus	Transmitted fecal-orally via contaminated food and water.	Watery diarrhea, vomiting, fever, stomach cramp.	[40]
Amoebiasis (amoebic dysentery)	*Entamoeba hystolitica*	Ingestion of faecally contaminated food and water containing amoebic cysts. Food involved include fruits, vegetables and drinking water.	Diarrhea, vomiting, dehydration, fever, headache, dizziness, insomnia, ulcer, drowsiness, weight loss, gastroenteritis.	[11]
Txoplsmosis	*Toxoplasma gondii*	Transmitted by taking vegetables containing the parasite.	Fever, headache, myalgia, rash	[41]
Taeniasis	*Taeniasaginata*, *Taeniasolium*	Transmitted vi eating fruits, vegetables, pork meat, beef meat that is contaminated with the pathogen.	Vomiting, diarrhea, insomnia, anorexia, weight loss, nervousness, gastroenteritis	[11]

Diseases	Pathogen	Mode of transmission and associated food	Clinical Manifestations	Reference
Ascariasis	*Ascarislimbriocoids*	ingestion of infective eggs from soil contaminated with feces or of contaminated vegetables and water	Vomiting, excretion of lived worms in the stool, indigestion, gastrointestinal discomfort.	[11]
Acute aflatoxicosis	*Aspergillusflavus*	Ingestion of aflatoxin in contaminated food such as milk, various cereals, oilseeds, spices, and nuts.	Nausea, vomiting, abdominal pain, convulsions, hepatotoxicity, immunotoxicity, and teratogenicity	[42]
Ochratoxicosis	*Aspergillus ochraceus*	Ingestion of food and water contaminated with ochratoxin A (OTA). Common food associated with OTA include but not limited to wine, beer, coffee, dried vine fruit, grape juices, pork, poultry, diary, spices, and chocolate	Loss of consciousness, fever, convulsion, inflammation of the liver, diarrhea.	[43]
Ergotism	*Clavisepspurpurea*	Transmitted via eating contaminated rye grass or by ergotamine orally.	Pains in the calf of the leg, swollen foot, mild diarrhea.	[30]

Table 1.
Common foodborne disease.

Common foodborne disease includes: botulism, cholera, gastroenteritis, intoxication, enteritis, listeriosis, shigellosis, typhoid, salmonellosis, dysentery, yersiniosis, amoebiasis, hepatitis A, viral gastroenteritis, bird flu, taxoplasmosis, taeniasis, ascariasis, aflatoxicosis, ergotism which are discussed in **Table 1.**

4. Mechanism of pathogenesis of foodborne pathogens

Microbial pathogenesis is a complex task that involves both the pathogens and the host, in this relationship, microbes are trying to gain into the host cell using their virulence factors such as flagella, pili, fimbriae, adhesins (adhesion proteins) e.g. fibronectin, collagen, laminin, integrin, internalin, and biofilm formation e.g. phospholipids, teichoic acids, nucleic acids, polysaccharides, proteins, capsules, enzymes, toxins, spikes, super antigens such as O, H, F, A, B antigens respectively [44]. on the other hand, host is trying to fight the effect of the pathogens using their immune cells such as gastric acids, mucus, bile salts, antimicrobial inhibitors, complement systems and phagocytic cells. At the end of the day, if the microbes succeeded, then the resultant effect is infection, while if the host immunity is strong the pathogens will be neutralized and they will eventually be killed [45].

Generally, foodborne microbes (virus, bacteria, fungi and/or parasites) get into the intestine through the mouth (oral route). Foodborne microbes cause variety of infections range from localized infection to general infection which can spread to almost all part of the body to caused systemic or generalized infection. Because the process is complex, for foodborne infection to be achieved, several factors must come together within the host. The process begins when the human ingests the pathogen in food or water that is contaminated with the pathogen, it will then eventually penetrate into the host cell in large quantity that can damage the host cell. As soon as it gains into the host cell, it then survives in the changing environment, multiply and propagate rapidly. After then, the pathogen colonizes the intestine using adhesive and invasive factors and chemotaxis respectively [46]. Several factors such as capsules, biofilm formation do protect the microbes to survive harsh environment, bacterial enzyme and toxins also safeguard the cells from eradication by the host immunity, certain commensals can also help the pathogen invade to find a suitable habitat for their growth and multiplication [47]. It is important to understand that most foodborne diseases attacked intestine, liver as a target size, thus resulting to liver damage and cancer in some cases can result to death. The pattern of pathogenesis by foodborne microbes is the same be it bacteria, virus, parasite, or fungi as it all started when the host ingest the pathogen in the faecally contaminated food or water, however, they mostly have the same target site; the intestine and the liver, that is why most of the resultant effect of the pathogenesis is gastroenteritis, liver damage and abdominal pain.

5. Conclusion

Foodborne microbial diseases are a significant public health threat. They occur in both developed and developing countries with different food industry expansion, food safety regulations, food hygiene and consumption habits, and climate and environmental situations should be considered as a preventive measure. The subsequent economic burden associated to them is also different. Most foodborne diseases are sporadic and often not reported, but sometimes foodborne outbreaks may affect a large number of individuals and compromise economic sectors and sanitary resources.

Acknowledgements

We would like to thank the authors and reviewers for their wonderful contributions and constructive criticisms to this special issue. We sincerely hope that this collection of papers will prompt further research and contribute to novel or improved strategies of foodborne pathogens- recent advances in control and detection to be able to further reduce the incidence of foodborne microbial diseases.

Author details

Ibrahim Musa Moi[1*], Zuhairu Ibrahim[1], Bashir Mohammed Abubakar[2], Yahaya Mohammed Katagum[3], Auwal Abdullahi[4], Gandi Ajibji Yiga[5], Badamasi Abdullahi[6], Ibrahim Mustapha[7], Jallaba Ali[7], Zinat Mahmud[4], Hamisu Maimusa[8], Halima Oge Katagum[9], Aisha Muhammad Malami[4], Aminu Mustapha[4] and Istifanus Ayuba[4]

1 Department of Microbiology, Bauchi State University, Bauchi, Nigeria

2 Department of Biological Sciences, Bauchi State University, Gadau, Bauchi, Nigeria

3 Department of Clinical Pharmacy and Pharmacy Administration, Bauchi State University, Gadau, Bauchi, Nigeria

4 Department of Microbiology, Bauchi State University, Gadau, Bauchi, Nigeria

5 Epidemiology Unit, Bauchi State Ministry of Health

6 Bill and Melinda Gates College of Health Technology, Ningi, Bauchi, Nigeria

7 Department of Medical Laboratory Science, College of Health Science and Technology, Nguru Yobe State, Nigeria

8 Department of Environmental Health Sciences, College of Health Science and Technology, Nguru Yobe State, Nigeria

9 Central Laboratory Complex, National Agency for Food and Drug Administration and Control (NAFDAC), Oshodi-Lagos, Nigeria

*Address all correspondence to: ibrahimmusamoi@gmail.com

IntechOpen

© 2022 The Author(s). Licensee IntechOpen. This chapter is distributed under the terms of the Creative Commons Attribution License (http://creativecommons.org/licenses/by/3.0), which permits unrestricted use, distribution, and reproduction in any medium, provided the original work is properly cited.

References

[1] Bintsis T. Foodborne pathogens. AIMS Microbiology. 2017;**3**(3):529

[2] Heredia N, García S. Animals as sources of food-borne pathogens: A review. Animal Nutrition. 2018;**4**(3):250-255

[3] Dhama K, Rajagunalan S, Chakraborty S, Verma AK, Kumar A, Tiwari R, et al. Food-borne pathogens of animal origin-diagnosis, prevention, control and their zoonotic significance: A review. Pakistan Journal of Biological Sciences: PJBS. 2013;**16**(20):1076-1085

[4] Bennett JW, Klich M. Mycotoxins. Clinical Microbiology Reviews. 2003;**16**: 497-516

[5] Albert MJ, Nair GB. *Vibrio cholerae*O139 Bengal-10 years on. Review in Medical Microbiology. 2005;**16**:135-143

[6] Brynestad S, Granum PE. *Clostridium perfringens* and foodborne infections. International Journal of Food Microbiology. 2002;**74**:195-202

[7] Li J, Adams V, Bannam TL, Miyamoto K, Garcia JP, Uzal FA, et al. Toxin plasmids of Clostridium perfringens. Microbiology and Molecular Biology Reviews. 2013;**77**(2):208-233

[8] Bohnel H, Gessler F. Botulinum toxins—Cause of botulism and systemic diseases? Veterinary Research Communications. 2005;**29**:313-345

[9] Bennett SD, Walsh KA, Gould LH. Foodborne disease outbreaks caused by *Bacillus cereus*, *Clostridium perfringens*, and *Staphylococcus aureus*—United States, 1998-2008. Clinical Infectious Diseases. 2013;**57**:425-433

[10] Bakardjiev AI, Theriot JA, Portnoy DA. *Listeria monocytogenes* traffics from maternal organs to the placenta and back. PLoS Pathogens. 2006;**2**:623-631

[11] Kayser FH. Basic Principles of medical microbiologie and immunology. 10th ed. ª 2005 Georg Thieme Verlag, Ru¨ digerstraße 14, 70469 Stuttgart, Germany

[12] Buchanan RL, Goris LGM, Hayman MM. A review of *Listeria monocytogenes*: An update on outbreaks, virulence, dose-response, ecology, and risk assessments. Food Control. 2017;**75**:1-13

[13] Dierick K, Coillie EV, Swiecicka I. Fatal family outbreak of *Bacillus cereus*-associated food poisoning. Journal of Clinical Microbiology. 2005;**43**: 4277-4279

[14] Baserisalehi M, Bahador N, Kapadnis BP. *Campylobacter:* An emerging pathogen. Research Journal of Microbiology. 2006;**1**:23-37

[15] Garcia A, Fox JG, Besser TE. Zoonotic enterohemorrhagic*Eschericia coli:* A one health perspective. ILAR Journal. 2010;**51**:221-232

[16] Beutin L. Emerging enterohaemorrhagic*Escherichia coli*, causes and effects of the rise of a human pathogen. Journal of Veterinary Medicine Series B. 2006;**53**:299-305

[17] Stewart GC. *Staphylococcus aureus*. In: Fratamico PM, Bhunia AK, Smith JL, editors. Foodborne Pathogens: Microbiology and Molecular Biology. Norfolk: Caister Academic; 2005. pp. 273-284

[18] Andrews HL, Baumler AJ. *Salmonella* species. In: Fratamico PM, Bhunia AK,

Smith JL, editors. Foodborne Pathogens: Microbiology and Molecular Biology. Norfolk: Caister Academic; 2005. pp. 327-339

[19] Zhang G, Ma L, Patel N. Isolation of *Salmonella* typhimurium from outbreak-associated cake mix. Journal of Food Protection. 2007;**70**:997-1001

[20] Vargas M, Gascon J, De Anta MTJ. Prevalence of Shigella enterotoxins 1 and 2 among Shigella strains isolated from patients with traveler's diarrhea. Journal of Clinical Microbiology. 1999;**37**:3608-3611

[21] Levine MM. Enteric infections and the vaccines to counter them: Future directions. Vaccine. 2006;**24**:3865-3873

[22] Longenberger AH, Gronostaj MP, Yee GY. *Yersinia enterocolitica* infections associated with improperly pasteurized milk products: Southwest Pennsylvania, March–August, 2011. Epidemiology and Infection. 2014;**142**:1640-1650

[23] Bhaduri S, Wesley IV, Bush EJ. Prevalence of pathogenic *Yersiniaenterocolitica*strains in pigs in the United States. Applied and Environmental Microbiology. 2005;**71**:7117-7121

[24] Dotzauer A. Encyclopedia of Virology. 3rd ed. Elsevier; 2008

[25] Cuthbert JA. Hepatitis A: Old and new. Clinical Microbiology Review. 2001;**14**:38-58

[26] Green KY, Balayan AT. Taxonomy of the calciviruses. The Journal of Infectious Diseases. 2000;**181**(Supplement 2): S322-S330

[27] Chhabra P, de Graaf M, Parra GI. Updated classification of norovirus genogroups and genotype. The Journal of General Virology. 2019;**100**(10):1393-1406

[28] Atmar RL, Estes MK. The epidemiologic and clinical importance of norovirus infection. Gastroenterology Clinics. 2006;**35**(2):275-290

[29] Estes MK, Prasad BV, Atmar RL. Noroviruses everywhere: Has something changed? Current Opinion in Infectious Diseases. 2006;**19**:467-474

[30] Cousin MA, Riley RT, Pestka JJ. Foodborne mycotoxins: Chemistry, biology, ecology, and toxicology. Foodborne Pathogen: Microbiology and Molecular Biology. 2005:163-226

[31] Janda JM, Brenden R, De Benedetti JA. Current perspectives on the epidemiology and pathogenesis of clinically significant *Vibrio* spp. Clinical Microbiology Review. 1988;**1**:245-267

[32] Grass JE, Gould LH, Mahon BE. Epidemiology of foodborne disease outbreaks caused by *Clostridium perfringens*, United States, 1998-2010. Foodborne Pathogens and Disease. 2013;**10**:131-136

[33] Carter AT, Peck MW. Genomes, neurotoxins and biology of *Clostridium botulinum* Group I and Group II. Research Microbiology. 2015;**166**:303-317

[34] Raheem D. Outbreaks of listeriosis associated with deli meats and cheese: An overview. AIMS Microbiology. 2016;**2**:230-250

[35] Rajkowski KT, Smith JL. Update: Food poisoning and other diseases induced by *Bacillus cereus*. In: Hui YH, Pierson MD, Gorham JR, editors. Foodborne Disease Handbook. New York: Markel Dekker, Inc; 2001. pp. 61-76

[36] Croxen MA, Law RJ, Scholz R. Recent advances in understanding enteric pathogenic *Escherichia coli*. Clinical Microbiology Review. 2013;**26**:822-880

[37] Cavallaro E, Date K, Medus C. *Salmonella* Typhimurium infections associated with peanut products. New England Journal of Medicine. 2011;**365**:601-610

[38] Hedberg CW, Levine WC, White KE. An international foodborne outbreak of Shigellosis associated with a commercial airline. JAMA. 1992;**268**:3208-3212

[39] Halliday ML, Lai LY, Zhou TK. An epidemic of Hepatitis A attributable to the ingestion of raw clams in Shanghai, China. The Journal of Infectious Diseases. 1991;**164**:852-859

[40] Glass RI, Parashar UD, Estes MK. Norovirus gastroenteritis. New England Journal of Medicine. 2009;**361**:1776-1785

[41] Bacon RT, Sofos JN. Characteristics of biological hazards in foods. In: Schmidt RH, Rodrick GE, editors. Food Safety Handbook. New Jersey: John Wiley & Sons, Inc; 2003. pp. 157-195

[42] Ngindu A, Kenya PR, Ocheng DM. Outbreak of acute hepatitis by aflatoxin poisoning in Kenya. Lancet. 2013;**319**:1346-1348. DOI: 10.1016/S0140-6736(82)92411-4

[43] Al-Alnati L, Petzinger E. Immunotoxic activity of ochratoxin A. Journal of Verterinary Pharmacology and Therapeutics. 2006;**29**(2):79-90

[44] Kazmierczak MJ, Wiedmann M, Boor KJ. Alternative sigma factors and their roles in bacterial virulence. Microbiology and Molecular Biology Reviews. 2005;**69**:527-543

[45] Galan JE, Collmer A. Type III secretion machines: Bacterial devices for protein delivery into host cells. Science. 1999;**284**:1322-1328

[46] Montecucco C, Papini E, Schiavo G. Bacterial protein toxins penetrate cells via a four-step mechanism. FEBS Letters. 1994;**346**:92-98

[47] Arun K. Mechanisms and Pathogenesis. 5th ed. New York: Springer Science+Business Media, LLC; 2008. pp. 130-171

Chapter 2

Emerging Infectious Food System Related Zoonotic Foodborne Disease – A Threat to Global Food Safety and Nutrition Security

Elechi Jasper Okoro Godwin, Vidhya Chandrasekaran, Adamu Cornelius Smah and Ekoja Omeyi Faith

Abstract

The zoonotic potential of foodborne infections, as well as their capacity to secrete toxins that cause a threat to global food safety and nutrition security and is enough to highlight the gravity of the problem. Feeding the estimated world population of 8.4–8.7 billion, 9.4–10.2 billion, and 11 billion people by 2030, 2050, and 2100, respectively, will require significant increases in crop and animal production, which will increase the agricultural use of antibiotics, water and pesticides and fertilisers, and contact between humans, wild and domestic animals, all of which will have implications for the emergence and spread of infectious agents. Hence, Infectious foodborne zoonotic illnesses are spreading at an unprecedented rate over the world. The evidence that animals are carriers of foodborne diseases is examined in this chapter. The processes through which infectious foodborne zoonosis impacts the global food and nutrition security, as well as how human infectious illnesses may affect food production and distribution are synthesised. The need for agricultural and disease management and policy activities, as well as a review of recent research on novel detection and control techniques in addressing the public health threat posed by foodborne Zoonotic illness, is also addressed.

Keywords: food safety, nutrition, foodborne infectious diseases, zoonosis, one health, emerging zoonotic disease, climate change, food system, animal health

1. Introduction

Agrifood systems cover the various dynamic and interconnected phases of agricultural production, processing, distribution, and consumption, with each phase including a variety of processes, value chains, numerous players, and their interactions [1]. In order to combat poverty, defend human rights, and restore ecosystems, the UN 2030 Agenda for Sustainable Development emphasises the importance of resilient agricultural methods and sustainable food production systems. A key component of such a system is food safety [1].

Foodborne zoonosis is an infectious disease brought on by consuming contaminated animal products. As a result, many bacteria, parasites and viruses that infect humans are present in vertebrate animals and are being spread through food on a regular basis. Foodborne bacterial infections have emerged long time ago and not related to environmental changes but other things related with food production and conservation. Environmental changes can be the cause of the appearance of new pathogens (emerging) coupled with increasing human susceptibility to sickness. The fight against foodborne bacterial diseases faces new challenges as a result of the constantly evolving human consumption patterns, the globalisation of the food industry, and climate change. Hence, infectious illnesses are emerging at an unprecedented rate, with serious consequences for the global economy and public health [2]. As a result, the social and economic aspects are of great importance. The social and environmental circumstances that contribute to the onset of illnesses, as well as management techniques that might lower the risk of emergence or recurrence, are of special interest [3, 4]. Malnutrition, defined as an insufficient intake of one or more nutrients, continues to be a major cause of disease globally [5]. Together, the extraordinary rate of infectious disease incidence and the need to feed the world population sustainably are two of the most daunting environmental and public health concerns of the twenty-first century [6], and they interact in complicated ways [4]. Access to safe, adequate, and nutritious food is an unquestionable human right [7, 8] and is critical for good health. A safe food supply benefits a country's economy, trade, and tourism, as well as food and nutrition security and sustainable development [9].

Emerging zoonotic diseases are those that are novel to human populations or that existed previously but are currently quickly growing in incidence or geographic range [10]. Fortunately, most of these infections are not fatal, and they do not spread widely. Some new illnesses, on the other hand, are having a significant influence. Ebola, HIV/AIDS, and, most recently, COVID-19 are well-known examples of new zoonoses that are especially harmful to human health and the economy [10]. Zoonoses have the potential to produce worldwide pandemics; historically, large-scale zoonotic epidemics resulting in high numbers of deaths caused major economic, political, and societal upheaval [11, 12]. People's interactions, both as merchants and consumers; the sale of live animals; food goods, especially ready-to-eat meals; and wild and peridomestic animals are all key risk factors for developing infectious illnesses [11]. These illnesses can be transmitted from animals to people if there is a barrier that permits infections to cross species, such as on a farm or at a market. Recent coronavirus (CoV) and avian influenza virus (AIV) outbreaks have convincingly proven that these emerging animal-borne zoonotic illnesses might constitute a hazard to human health [11, 13].

In the EU each year there are more than 200,000 cases of Campylobacteriosis and more than 50,000 of Salmonellosis. According to EFSA [14] report, "campylobacteriosis and salmonellosis were respectively the first and second most reported zoonoses in humans in 2020. Yersiniosis was the third most reported zoonosis in humans, with 10-foldless cases reported than salmonellosis, followed by Shiga toxin-producing *Escherichia coli* (STEC) and *Listeria monocytogenes* infections. Illnesses caused by *L. monocytogenes* and West Nile virus infections were the most severe zoonotic diseases with the highest case fatality". In India, animal products are responsible for around 70% of foodborne diseases [15]. The three types of foodborne diseases are intoxification (a toxin produced by pathogens that cause foodborne illness), infection (ingestion of pathogen-containing food), and toxicoinfections (production of toxins during growth in the human gut) [16–18]. Human-animal infections can be spread by direct touch, indirect environmental contact, and/or food intake [19]. Approximately 60% of human illnesses are caused by animals, and approximately 75% of emerging human infectious diseases are passed from vertebrates to humans [20].

Many viruses that cause human illness after being transferred through food are naturally found in vertebrate animals [21]. Humans are exposed to pathogenic bacteria through three different food sources: meat (beef, mutton, and pork), dairy (milk, cheese, yoghurt, and ice cream), and eggs [22]. Environmental difficulties have resulted in the emergence of foodborne bacterial pathogens and increased human vulnerability to illness [23]. Due to rapidly changing human consumption habits, food market globalisation, and climate change, the battle against foodborne bacterial infections confronts new problems [16, 24]. The purpose of this chapter focuses:

I. The evidence that animals are carriers of foodborne diseases

II. The ways through which infectious foodborne zoonoses undermine global food and nutrition security.

III. The impact of human infectious illnesses on food production and distribution.

IV. The importance of agricultural and disease-related interventions, as well as political actions.

V. A review of recent research on innovative detection and control approaches for foodborne zoonotic illnesses, which constitute a public health danger.

2. Why diseases emerge and the wicked problem

Zoonoses transferred from animal hosts to humans have evolved in food systems as a result of a lack of food safety monitoring and enforcement [25]. In regulated production systems and wildlife trafficking, improper animal storage, filthy environments, and poor handling of animal products have been identified as pathways for viral strain mutation and interspecies transmission [12, 26–28]. Viruses such as the new coronavirus have found an opportunity to spread into pandemics, aided by human-to-human transmission due to urbanisation, increased ease of local and worldwide transit, and growing antibiotic resistance [29, 30].

King [31] assessed the convergence of conditions contributing to the global rise of foodborne illnesses. The variety of global food safety issues and their causes describes disease onset as a perfect microbial storm, according to the convergence model of variables influencing the establishment of infectious illnesses [32]. **Table 1** depict the numerous elements that impact the complex host-pathogen-environment interactions that can result in the formation or recurrence of infectious illnesses [32, 34]. Zoonoses arise through a complicated process. A variety of external causes or drivers generate the circumstances for a disease to expand and adapt to a new habitat. The primary motivators include environmental, political, economic, and social pressures at the local, national, regional, and global levels. Hotspots for zoonotic diseases are areas where these characteristics are most densely aggregated, common, and where the likelihood of a disease outbreak is greatest [35].

Genetic and biological factors	Physical environmental factors	Ecological factors	Social, political, and economic factors
• Microbial adaptation and change	• Climate and weather	• Changing ecosystems	• International travel and commerce
• Human susceptibility to infection	• Economic development and land use	• Human demographics and behaviour	• Poverty and social inequity
			• War and famine
			• Lack of political will
			• Intent to harm

Source: King [31], Choffnes et al. [33].

Table 1.
Factors influencing the emergence or Reemergence of infectious diseases.

Several environmental elements, including but not limited to the following [33], are particularly important for the establishment and transmission of foodborne infections:

- **Intensive farming methods.** Raising and moving big herds of cattle, flocks of birds, or shoals of fish or shellfish in close quarters in the quest of efficiency creates perfect circumstances for the onset and spread of illness [36].

- **Increased interactions between humans, domestic animals, and wildlife.** Increased interaction between humans, animals, and their associated microorganisms, sometimes induced by habitat degradation, changing land-use patterns, and killing of animals for food or the food trade, further increases the possibility for disease transmission across animal species or between humans and animals [37].

- **Environmental "commons" such as water.** Contamination of shared resources disperses and raises the danger of pathogen and chemical contaminant emergence, and it can spread across farms, regions, states, and countries.

Jones et al. [3] stated that significant emerging viral illnesses such as HIV/AIDS and severe acute respiratory syndrome (SARS) are classified as foodborne pathogens since their entrance into humans and subsequent transmission is intimately tied to food availability. This includes a huge variety of viruses that have spread from wild or cattle populations to individuals who seek bushmeat (HIV/AIDS) or kill and process exotic and domesticated animals in wet markets [38]. The killing and percutaneous and mucosal contact with blood and body fluids of non-human primates hunted in Sub-Saharan Africa are most likely linked to the spread of HIV and Ebola hemorrhagic fever.

King [31] introduced the concept of the "wicked problem," and demonstrated why the hunt for safe food in a globalised world matches this criterion. According to King, [31], wickedness refers to the inability of such issues to be treated by normal techniques to maintaining food safety, which are based on medical education and training concepts that aim to describe a problem, make a diagnosis, and prescribe a remedy. The researcher promotes the One Health concept, which acknowledges the interconnection of humans, animals, and the environment and stresses illness prevention as a means of solving these difficult and emerging problems [33].

3. Animals: carriers of foodborne diseases

Zoonotic infections can be spread both by Animal Sources Food (ASF) and by non-ASF that get infected during the manufacturing process [39]. One study found that over 60% of emerging human infectious diseases are zoonotic, with the majority (72%) of these being of wild animal origin [3], while another estimate suggested that 75% of emerging pathogens were zoonotic [40], putting ASF consumers at risk [41]. While estimates vary, most new viruses are thought to originate in animals. Many new epizootic and zoonotic viral infections contain single-stranded RNA viruses like coronaviruses, which can cause serious infections in both animals and humans [11]. 1445 novel RNA viruses have recently been identified in Invertebrates while over 200 previously undiscovered viruses have been discovered in vertebrates [42, 43]. Food-producing animals (e.g., cattle, chickens, pigs, and turkeys) are the primary reservoirs for several foodborne infections, including *Campylobacter spp., Salmonella enterica* or non-Typhi serotypes, *E. coli* Shiga toxin-producing strains, and *L. monocytogenes* [44]. *Salmonella* is found in both domestic and wild animals, including cats, dogs, amphibians, reptiles, and rodents [44].

Poultry is thought to be the primary source of *Campylobacter* species transfer to humans [45], owing to their higher body temperature. Handling, processing, and consumption of chicken meat can account for 20–30% of human campylobacteriosis infections, whereas the chicken reservoir as a whole accounts for 50–80% [46]. Campylobacteriosis has also been related to cattle dogs, pigs, and piglets [44, 45]. In addition to the concerns already mentioned, contact with pets is another potential source of human illness [47].

Cattle and other ruminants are assumed to be the principal reservoirs of Shiga toxin-producing E. coli (STEC) [44]. *L. monocytogenes* has been recovered from cattle, sheep, goats, and poultry, primarily on their skin, although several studies have shown that this bacterium is also found in muscle, albeit at low levels [48]. Crustaceans, shellfish, molluscs, and related goods, cheese, meat and meat products, pork and related products, vegetables, juices, and related items such as mixed salads and soft cheese are all food carriers for *L. monocytogenes* [48].

4. Changing food system and foodborne zoonotic diseases

Rohr et al. [4] and Tilman et al. [49] reported that deficiency of nutrients is expected to worsen as climate change occurs. According to the United Nations, the world population will expand by over 4 billion to more than 11 billion people by 2100 [50]. Achieving the United Nations Sustainable Development Goal of eliminating hunger for the world's rising population would necessitate a significant increase in food supply, as well as significant changes in agricultural production and distribution systems, infrastructure, and social protection programs [4, 51, 52]. Historically, increased wealth has been correlated with higher food consumption in general and animal-based food consumption in particular, both of which further increase food demand and the need for agricultural expansion or intensification [4, 53]. Recent studies have shown that agricultural production may need to double or triple by 2100 in order to keep up with the global economy and keep pace with projected population growth and demand for food [4, 51, 52, 54]. Agriculture currently uses more than two-thirds of the world's freshwater and occupies about half of the world's land area [55]. Despite ongoing advancements in agricultural efficiency, a reevaluation of these estimates will be necessary. In order to meet these needs with current agricultural production systems, it may be necessary to replace more than 109 hectares of natural ecosystems with agricultural production. According to estimates by Foley et al. [51], Tilman et al. [49], and Rohr et al. [4], this rise in agriculture might also result in an estimated 2-fold increase in irrigation, a 2.7-fold increase in fertiliser, and a 10-fold increase in pesticide usage.

There are various ways in which the problems of feeding more than 11 billion people and controlling infectious illnesses are related [4]. First, tropical developing countries are experiencing disproportionate agricultural expansion and intensification [51] in which infectious diseases account for 75% of deaths [56] and the risk of disease emergence is highest, and where disease surveillance and access to health care, particularly for those infections associated with extreme poverty, are most restricted [3]. Second, historically significant habitat change, pollution with animal waste, and greater use of agricultural inputs like pesticides and antibiotic growth promoters have all occurred in conjunction with agricultural expansion and intensification [4]. Aside from their direct detrimental effects on human health [57], agricultural biochemical inputs are known to have an indirect driving force in the emergence of wildlife diseases [4, 58], which are significant sources of emerging human infections [3, 30], as well as direct effects on human infectious diseases. The improvement of diet, however, has demonstrable advantages in reducing the prevalence of many infectious illnesses at the individual and population levels [5, 59].

4.1 Food system transition and animal health

In order to achieve crucial global goals at the junction of human and planetary well-being, there is widespread agreement that food systems must be transformed [51, 60]. Therefore, in order to cultivate agrifood systems that are resilient, sustainable, and equitable in the face of economic, social, and environmental challenges, there are growing efforts underway to transform agrifood systems so that the expanding global population has access to food that is nourishing, safe, and affordable [1]. Giving everyone access to more nutrient-dense meals is vital, and hence, future food systems must offer a wide variety of reasonably priced foods to enable everyone to have access to diets of high nutritional quality. To ensure that the circumstances that have made it possible for people to survive on the planet and the present Earth's ecosystems to flourish continue, a significant reduction in the ecological footprint of the livestock sector is required [60].

4.2 Animal husbandry intensification and veterinary drugs abuses

The cost of cattle products has grown as a result of the Westernisation of diets and the rise in demand for nutritional diversity in many emerging nations [61]. Animal production has increased, gaining from agricultural industry's economies of scale [62]. The genetic variety of cattle breeds has been decreased as productivity has been increased to preserve competitiveness in livestock production systems. Antimicrobial resistance in people has been reported to rise when antibiotics are overused in livestock production to promote growth and maintain herd health [25]. Agribusiness uses a larger portion of the world's antibiotic and anthelmintic production than human medicine to prevent catastrophic disease-related losses and enhance animal growth. The majority of antibiotics are given in non-therapeutic doses because there is no known disease [63, 64]. Although estimates are lacking for the majority of the nations in the world, in the United States, animals receive about nine times as many antibiotics as people do, and of those given to animals, more than 12 times as many are used for non-therapeutic purposes than for therapeutic ones [63]. Given that it appears to encourage microbial resistance to these medications, some of which are also used in human medicine, the widespread use of antibiotics and antiparasitics (such as anthelmintics) in industrialised agriculture and aquaculture could have significant effects on infectious diseases affecting humans [63]. For instance, antibiotic-resistant strains of *Salmonella, Campylobacter*, and *E. coli* are that are harmful to humans are mostly found in cattle [63]. There is proof that bacteria with antibiotic resistance genes acquired from aquaculture can spread to human systems and cause epidemics [4]. According to Rohr et al. [4] anthelmintic resistance is common among parasitic worms that infest animals and is significantly associated with human parasite worms. It is likely that current antibiotics and anthelmintics will lose some of their effectiveness due to developed resistance as animal and aquaculture production increases to meet rising food needs [64]. This will make treating infectious diseases in domestic animals and humans more challenging. There are now worries that insufficient antibiotic usage in cattle would create antimicrobial resistance, harming human health and undermining human antimicrobial therapy.

4.3 Climate change and food borne zoonotic disease

Food value chains have a detrimental influence on the environment since they require energy, raw materials, and modify how land is used [65]. The frequency, severity, and unpredictability of extreme events linked to climate change are increasing. In addition to negatively influencing agricultural productivity and yield and upsetting supply systems, such catastrophes also have an influence on food safety [1]. Increased temperatures have a serious impact on various biological and chemical contaminants in food by changing their virulence, occurrence, and distribution [1]. Other factors include the alternation of severe drought periods and heavy rains, soil quality degradation, rising sea levels, and ocean acidification. Due to this, more people are at risk of contracting foodborne illnesses. Additionally, the increased globalisation of the food supply chains makes it easier for foodborne dangers to spread along the route, creating potential for local outbreaks of foodborne illness to become international outbreaks [1].

It is predictable that climate change would hasten the spread of vector-borne illnesses (such those carried by flies), including those that are food-borne pathogens [65]. On the other hand, the adverse higher temperatures might stress fisheries and livestock, increasing their susceptibility to diseases and causing diseased animals to moult more frequently [9]. (**Figure 1**). More frequent flooding and rain events will enable the spread of infections and chemical risks through runoff in agricultural regions, leaving cropland vulnerable [9, 66]. The deterioration of water quality for drinking and agriculture has also been connected to these catastrophes. On the other side, unfavourable higher temperatures can have an impact on fisheries and cattle health. In addition to infections and increased animal disease shedding, livestock are also susceptible to dietary shortages and animal disease outbreaks (**Figure 1**) [9]. As a result, these occurrences will increase the danger to food safety [67]. For instance,

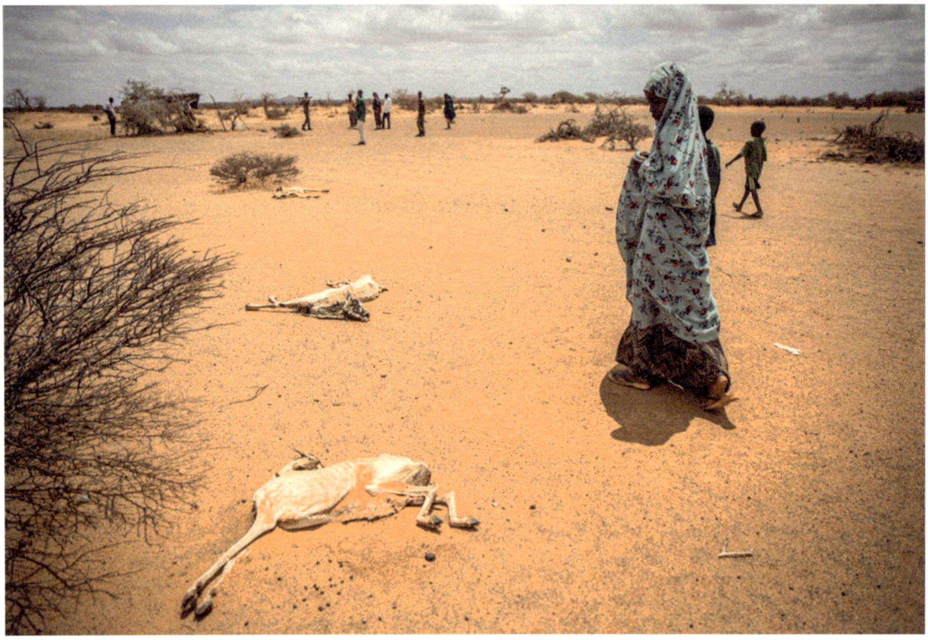

Figure 1.
A child walks past goats that died from hunger and thirst outside Dollow, Somalia, on April 14, 2022. Sally Hayden/SOPA images/LightRocket/Getty. Source: Global Health NOW Johns Hopkins Bloomberg School of Public Health Issue No. 2085 June 9, 2022.

deforestation brings about the introduction of new animal species that are carriers of disease vectors and are generally hazardous to human health [30, 68]. Long-term climate change also presents difficulties for the resurgence of infectious illnesses that have been eradicated due to shifting ecological habitats [69]. The loss of biodiversity and climate change have increased the new risks posed by these illnesses.

E. coli, a bacteria that causes gastroenteritis, is virulent, and its virulence is strongly connected with both temperature and precipitation. Due to the introduction of novel pathogens and vectors into temperate zones as well as temperature-related changes in contamination levels, climate change also results in a rise in foodborne illnesses [25, 70]. Rapid urbanisation, intensification of animal production, modernisation of food marketing systems, and changes in food consumption patterns have caused ecosystem degradation [21]. New zoonotic infections are emerging as a result of some of these conditions, while endemic zoonoses are reemerging as a result of others [41]. Eutrophication and acidification of water bodies are two additional environmental effects that modify aquatic ecosystems and their ecological resilience [71]. As a result, these occurrences will increase the danger to food safety [67].

5. Emerging infectious foodborne zoonotic disease

The most recent and dramatic example of the possible establishment of zoonoses in human populations is the suspected emergence of the SARS-CoV2 virus from an unknown animal source in or near the Wuhan Seafood Market in late 2019 [41]. The COVID-19 pandemic, if proven true, will be one of the most prominent instances of zoonotic spillover in recent memory, following the relatively recent emergence of the severe acute respiratory syndrome (SARS), Middle East respiratory syndrome (MERS), Nipah virus, swine flu, and highly pathogenic avian influenza (H5N1) [72].

The origin and spread of COVIDs from their origins in an unofficial wet market clearly demonstrate that comparable foodborne dangers might be enhanced by such attitudes [41]. Its cascading effects and disruption of local food systems in Low- and Medium-Income Countries (LMICs) highlight how difficult it is to prevent and manage the spread of such pathogens internationally [73].

5.1 *Campylobacter spp*

Campylobacter spp. is the world's most common source of zoonotic enteric infections and a contributor to foodborne diseases. Human campylobacter infections are mostly spread via the food chain [74]. *Campylobacter (C.) jejuni*, one of the *Campylobacter spp.*, is the most common cause of bacterial food-borne gastroenteritis globally with more than 96 million cases annually [75, 76]. The lower digestive tract of many animals often harbours these bacteria asymptomatically. *Campylobacter jejuni*, however, when infects people, it can lead to significant illness states [77, 78]. Consuming inadequately cooked chicken meat is the main way for the bacteria to spread to humans. Usually in healthy people, *C. jejuni* infections can last up to 2 weeks and are self-limiting, but problems are more common in kids, the elderly, or those with impaired immune systems [76].

5.2 Salmonellosis

One of the most often reported foodborne zoonoses is salmonellosis [79, 80]. From farm to fork, the causative agent, Salmonella can be transferred to people, mainly through contaminated food with an animal origin [81]. Globally, Salmonella spp. is thought to be responsible for 155,000 fatalities and 93.8 million instances of acute gastroenteritis [82, 83]. According to the Centers for Disease Control and Prevention (CDC), Salmonella spp. results in 1.2 million illnesses, 23,000 hospitalizations, and 450 fatalities annually in the United States, costing an estimated $400 million in direct medical expenditures that would otherwise be incurred [80]. While Salmonella spp. caused 43% of foodborne outbreaks in the United States in 2018 [81, 82], they were responsible for 24.4% of all foodborne outbreaks in Europe in 2016 [79, 80].

5.3 *Listeria*

The bacterium listeria is typically found in soil, surface water, plants, and food. It is spread by a wide range of animals. Along with people, *Listeria* can also be found in at least 42 other types of wild and domesticated mammals and 17 different types of birds, including domestic and wild poultry. *Listeria* have been found in oysters, fish, crabs, ticks, and flies [33]. Infected animals can shed the pathogen through their faeces, milk, and uterine secretions, which is how most infections are contracted [84]. The relatively uncommon but hazardous disease listeriosis, which has a mortality rate of about 20% in humans, can be brought on by listeria infection [33]. According to Scallan et al. [85]'s estimate, *Listeria monocytogenes* causes 255 fatalities, 1455 hospitalizations, and an average of 1591 incidents of domestically acquired foodborne disease per year in the United States [85]. For instance, the world's greatest epidemic of listeriosis occurred in South Africa between 2018 and 2019, resulting in more than 1000 laboratory-confirmed cases and more than 200 fatalities among those who caught the disease after consuming contaminated food [10, 86]. Listeria is highly suited to conditions of food preparation and storage. At low refrigeration temperatures, it can proliferate and cause lingering infections on food processing equipment [87]. After being cleaned and sanitised, *L. monocytogenes* can develop in biofilms that shield them from environmental stress [87].

5.4 *Escherichia coli*

E. coli is a vast and varied genus of bacteria that may be found in the environment and in a range of animals, including humans, as commensal organisms [88]. *E. coli* that produces the shiga toxin (STEC) is one of the most infamous foodborne pathogens. Hemolytic uremic syndrome (HUS), a hazardous consequence marked by copious bleeding that can result in kidney failure and death, develops in 5–10% of infections caused by STEC, and it can cause mild to severe diarrhoea [89]. According to estimates by Scallan et al. [85], STEC strain O157:H7 results in 63,000 infections, 2100 hospitalizations, and 20 fatalities annually. The digestive system of cattle is the primary reservoir for this zoonotic infection.

5.5 *Brucella spp*

The bacterium genus Brucella is the source of the zoonotic illness known as brucellosis. By ingesting contaminated food items, coming into close contact with sick animals, or inhaling aerosols, the germs can be transferred from animals to people. The illness is widespread and has several names, including undulant fever, Mediterranean fever, Malta fever, and remitting stomach fever mostly transmitted to humans by raw milk or close contact with sick animals. Human infections cause a fluctuating temperature, joint discomfort, and weakness [90].

5.6 Cryptosporidiosis

Cryptosporidiosis is a diarrheal disease mostly severs on young animals and children and immunocompromised adults. Among 44 species 21 are reported with human infection but *C. hominis* and *C. parvum* are most frequently found in intestinal infections with symptoms of watery diarrhoea, pain, abdominal cramps, vomiting, nausea, dehydration, fever, and weight loss are most symptoms associated with cryptosporidiosis [91]. The food sources include shellfish, uncooked beef, pork, and chicken.

5.7 *Mycobacterium bovis*

Raw milk is the main channel of *M. bovis* transmission from cattle to people. The signs and symptoms of *Mycobacterium tuberculosis* are same in humans. Africa is thought to have the largest incidence of zoonotic tuberculosis (TB), due to the prevalence in cattle and the absence of pasteurisation in the majority of milk drank there [92].

5.8 *Toxoplasma gondii*

Toxoplasma gondii is one of the most pervasive zoonoses. Humans get the disease through consuming cysts in raw meat or by coming into touch with food and water contaminated by the sporulated oocysts of cats, the disease's ultimate host. Although toxoplasmosis is often asymptomatic, foetuses, the elderly, and those with impaired immune systems are especially vulnerable. [41, 93].

5.9 *Taenia solium*

The parasitic zoonoses *Theridion solium* use pigs as their intermediate host. Consuming pork that is not fully cooked causes tapeworm (taeniosis) infection at its most advanced stage. Following faecal-oral transmission in humans, neurocysticercosis, a prominent cause of epilepsy in endemic places, can result from an aberrant intermediate-stage infection [41, 93].

5.10 Fish borne trematodes

Fish muscles contain *metecercaiae*, which when ingested by humans can lead to cholangitis, pancreatitis, and chronic liver disease in some people [21].

5.11 *Paragonimus spp*

This zoonotic parasite infects humans when they consume raw or undercooked seafood. Flukes that are still developing go to the lungs, where they cause inflammation-related pulmonary symptoms. The parasite is particularly common in Asia, where eating raw shellfish is a cultural habit that supports the parasite's life cycle [94].

5.12 *Trichinellosis*

Trichinellosis is a dangerous and occasionally deadly human illness that is caused by parasitic nematodes of the genus *Trichinella*. *Trichinella* larvae are transmitted to humans through the consumption of inadequately prepared meat. It has traditionally been linked to the intake of pig meat [95]. According to Rostami et al. [96], wild boar meat is presently the second most significant source of human trichinellosis and has been linked to several human outbreaks in Europe. Trichinellosis severity mostly relies on the quantity of larvae consumed (the infectious dosage), how frequently contaminated meat is consumed [97].

5.13 Hepatitis E virus

According to Hoofnagle et al. [98] Hepatitis E virus (HEV) the responsible agent, has been genetically linked to humans as well as a number of other animal species [99, 100]. Pigs and maybe other animal species serve as HEV reservoirs, and hepatitis E is now regarded as a zoonotic disease [99]. Concerns about zoonotic diseases and food safety have been raised by occasional and cumulative instances of acute hepatitis E being linked to direct contact with diseased animals and eating of tainted animal meat and meat products [100]. HEV genotypes 1 (G1) and 2 (G2) were estimated to cause 20 million yearly infections in 2005 [101, 102]. HEV typically results in an acute, self-limiting infection that goes away in a few weeks, but in some people (such as those with compromised immune systems), these infections can become chronic, lead to acute liver failure known as fulminant hepatitis, or have extrahepatic manifestations, which can be fatal [101].

5.14 Monkeypox virus

While clinically less severe than smallpox, monkeypox is a viral zoonosis with symptoms that are comparable to those experienced by historical smallpox victims. Primarily occurring in central and western Africa, monkeypox is increasingly common in cities and frequently found close to tropical rainforests. Direct contact with blood, bodily fluids, or skin or mucosal lesions of infected animals can result in animal-to-human transmission (zoonosis) [103]. Numerous animals in Africa, including rope squirrels, tree squirrels, Gambian opossums, dormice, numerous monkey species, and others, have shown signs of infection with the monkeypox virus. A potential risk factor is consuming raw meat and other animal products from infected animals [103]. According to a WHO estimate, the monkeypox epidemic in 2022 is on the verge of becoming a global public health emergency (PHEIC) with more than 6000 cases reported in 58 countries. More than 80% of the cases in the ongoing outbreak in 2022 are in Europe.

5.15 Nipah virus

The spread of the Nipah virus (NiV) in Malaysia and Bangladesh is a particularly lethal illustration of the various channels via which zoonotic diseases are transmitted and how these channels are connected to the food chain [33]. Flying foxes of the genus *Pteropus* serve as the paramyxovirus's primary reservoir in animals [104]. Nipah virus was initially identified as the result of a Malaysian outbreak in 1999, but it is now more frequently linked to Bangladesh and the surrounding regions of India, where multiple outbreaks over the past decade have led to more than 250 cases and nearly 200 fatalities, according to Luby et al. [105]. According to Epstein et al. [106] and Choffnes et al. [33], the Malaysian outbreak, which has killed more than 100 people and infected about 40% of those who have been identified, was initially linked to close contact with infected pigs. However, it has since been determined that infected bats that reside in forested areas close to large-scale commercial pig farms were likely the source of the outbreak.

5.16 Influenza

Avian influenza viruses (AIV) are classified as types A, B, C, or D based on genetic variations and are members of the *Orthomyxoviridae* family [107]. The influenza A virus is naturally found in birds, where it can spread to people and cause zoonotic diseases [108]. Direct contact with infected birds, eating raw or undercooked chicken products, and human-to-human transmission are all risk factors for human infections [109]. Growing international trade (including live bird markets) and wild bird movement are factors in the development of the illness [107]. According to Libera et al. [107], a human infection can present as a mild upper respiratory tract infection that causes fever, headache, and cough in addition to conjunctivitis and digestive issues. However, acute respiratory distress, multiple organ failure, shock, and severe pneumonia can develop quickly [110]. Viruses generated from HPAI A (H5N1) and LPAI A (H7N9) infections are responsible for the most deadly illnesses in humans [111].

The influenza A virus (IAV), generally known as the swine flu virus, is what causes swine flu (SIV). Hemagglutinin (HA) and neuraminidase (NA), two proteins, are used to categorise IAVs into 18H and 11 N subtypes [110]. The (H1N1) pdm09 novel triple reassortant virus, one of the IAVs, produced a pandemic in the human population in 2009 [107]. IAVs may infect both pigs and people. In both people and pigs, symptoms include respiratory system (sneezing, coughing, and trouble breathing), fever, tiredness, and reduced appetite [112].

5.17 Severe acute respiratory syndrome (SARS)

The coronavirus known as SARS-CoV, which causes SARS, was originally discovered in China in February 2003 and presumably originated in bats [10]. It then likely moved to other species (mainly civet cats), and finally to people. This pneumonia-like sickness spread to more than a dozen nations in North America, South America, Europe, and Asia. Horseshoe bats have been shown to have a coronavirus that resembles SARS, indicating that bats are natural reservoirs [10]. Since 2004 there have been no cases documented [113].

5.18 Ebola

According to Knipe et al. [114], the Ebola virus disease (EVD) is one of the deadliest viral infections that may afflict both people and monkeys. The *Rhabdoviridae* and *Paramyxoviridae* families of viruses, which also contain the Ebola virus (EV), are members of the order *Mononegavirales*. This pandemic illness is marked by hemorrhagic symptoms that can cause shock, organ failure, and mortality [115]. It also causes fever, intense weariness, and joint discomfort. It spreads to people by skin-to-skin contact or body fluids exuded by infected animals including fruit bats, chimps, and monkeys. A major source of oral Ebola virus transmission, particularly in African nations, is eating raw contaminated meat like bat or chimpanzee [116].

Hunters who opportunistically shot and processed sick gorilla and chimpanzee carcasses for meat consumption spread the disease in Central Africa [10, 117]. While there is a danger associated with eating game meat without following minimal hygienic requirements, it is not the only factor. Secondary epidemiological cycles are involved in the largest Ebola outbreaks in West Africa and the eastern DRC at present, highlighting the fact that human conditions and actions, not unintentional transmission effects, are the main determinant in zoonoses' spread [10].

5.19 Lassa fever

This foodborne zoonosis, Lassa fever, was found and named after a town in Nigeria and causes significant health and food safety issues in Africa. *Mastomys natalensis*, a common type of rat, transmits the lassa virus, which is excreted in faeces and urine. Human infection results through ingesting contaminated food and drink or from coming into direct touch with infected items and open skin sores. Inhaling airborne particles from actions like sweeping or touching the rodent while it is being prepared for consumption are other ways in which contamination might occur. Contact with an infected person's body fluids can result in human-to-human transmission. For instance, 58 million people in West Africa are at risk, with 100,000 to 300,000 suspected cases of Lassa fever and 5000 suspected fatalities per year [118].

6. Infectious foodborne zoonoses and impact mechanisms on global food safety and nutrition security

Recent years have seen the development of sophisticated and efficient methods for foodborne zoonotic agents to transmit diseases from animals to people [119]. Poverty and food instability have been the root causes of epidemics like Ebola and HIV, and rising demand for wildlife for commerce and consumption has increased human-wildlife interaction [120]. Mechanism through which foodborne zoonoses impact global system food safety and nutrition security have to be examined.

6.1 Food losses and waste

Over 14% of food produced worldwide is lost before it leaves the field, and 17% of food that is available to customers is wasted in stores and homes [121, 122]. According to Tilman et al. [49], in the past 25 years alone, outbreaks of foot-and-mouth disease and the influenza A virus (H5N1) have killed more than 1.2 million chickens and 6 million animals in China and Great Britain, respectively. Mad cow disease has also resulted in the slaughter of 11 million cattle globally. The highly infectious avian influenza virus strain has also been discovered in overcrowded chicken farms in Thailand and Vietnam [123]. Vietnam and Thailand paid about $45 million and $135 million, respectively, to contain the epidemic. Food supplies were devastated by the epidemic. In order to control the epidemic, over 18% of the entire chicken population in Vietnam and 15% of the total poultry population in Thailand were slaughtered in 2004 [124]. Similar situations have happened in aquaculture, particularly in impoverished nations with poor hygiene.

6.2 Reduction in optimal nutrition/dietary intake

Development in agriculture may directly enhance nutrition, and nutrition can influence infectious disease susceptibility and progression via a number of pathways [125]. By raising the body's requirement for nutrients when sick reduced food intake, malabsorption, and metabolic losses of nutrients, infection can lead to malnutrition [126]. Fear of contracting a foodborne disease can deter consumers from purchasing or consuming ASPs in both high- and low-income contexts [127–129]. Due to a lack of alternatives, consumers in nations where the aforementioned foods are unavailable either increase their risk of developing food-borne diseases by consuming the foods or they raise their risk of malnutrition by excluding nutritious foods from their diets [130]. For instance, after the avian influenza epidemic in Egypt in 2006, a surge in human stunting was seen as a result of the decreased poultry availability (and less dietary variety) brought on by the widespread slaughter of poultry to suppress the outbreak [131]. As malnourished people become more prone to infections, such dynamics can result in a vicious cycle of undernutrition and illness [130]. Because many parasite illnesses exert direct demands on host nutrition, undernutrition can result when food is scarce [132]. Even eating disorders like geophagy (the desire to eat earth), bulimia, and anorexia can be brought on by certain parasites, such as helminths [133]. Persistence infections frequently need quick and efficient tissue healing, which is also expensive.

6.3 Human infectious illnesses impact food production and distribution

The economic and agricultural growth required to feed the expanding human population can also be impacted by human infectious illnesses [4]. Zoonotic illnesses pose a hazard to human health and well-being, animal health and production, and consumer health [134]. According to estimates by Grace et al. [135], zoonotic illnesses and diseases that have recently originated from animals account for more than a quarter of the disability-adjusted life years (DALYs) lost to infectious diseases in low-income nations like sub-Saharan Africa. Areas with higher historical tsetse-fly abundance, the vector of the parasite (*Trypanosoma brucei*) that causes African sleeping sickness in humans and cattle, experienced greater lags in the adoption of animal husbandry practices that hindered agricultural development and prosperity in Africa long before and after Europeans colonised [4, 136]. In rural subsistence communities, any source of ill health can significantly impact people's productivity, yields and agricultural output [137]. For instance, since 1997, the human immunodeficiency virus/AIDS has reduced the average life expectancy in sub-Saharan Africa by 5 years. Some low-income populations appear to be stuck in the poverty-disease cycle, and as a result, they may need significant health system financing to support the crucial agricultural and economic growth that will help break the pattern [137, 138].

7. Food system approaches to control of foodborne zoonotic diseases

The main goal of food systems is to provide safe and nourishing food for people, with the ultimate goals being nutrition and fitness. Food safety refers to the circumstances and procedures applied to the food system in order to prevent foodborne disease and minimise serious health risks [130]. Pathogen prevention and control methods are not always easy. However, Sahoo et al. [139] state that the following crucial steps must be put into place in farms and processing facilities since they can be effective in lowering the risk of infection: (1) Clean management procedures and separating sick animals from healthy ones, (2) safety measures at both the farm and processing levels, (3) well-planned precautions, such as animal testing, full-size homes, and wild animals vaccination, (4) cooling after animal slaughter, (5) animal health training, (6) Use of antibiotics and phytonutrient-rich feed, (7) modern food processing techniques, (8) adequate kitchen cleaning, cooking, and sanitization procedures, (9) avoiding cross-contamination and ingestion of raw or undercooked animal products, and (10) routine product inspection, monitoring, and sampling.

7.1 Man-Imal: from animal to man one health strategies

In a globalised, industrialised society with an increasing number of stakeholders and regulations, production chains are becoming more and more complex. Based on the "One World, One Health" concept promoted by the WHO, FAO and OIE, the '*man-imal*' (From Animal to Man) seek to engage multidisciplinary approach in "Analysing and Managing Health and Food Risks" as being anchored by "Oniris" a French institution. Hence, the success of One Health (formerly One Medicine) initiatives will provide the foundation for advancements in food safety, public health, and welfare in the future decades. The key tenet of this concept is that there is a close relationship and interdependence between the environment and both human and animal health [107]. One Health is an all-encompassing or comprehensive approach where the assumption is that welfare and wellbeing are founded on human, animal, and environmental health and that integration and exchange of information on animal and human health is the key to effective health systems [140]. For tackling complicated health issues, One Health represents a rapidly expanding variety of synergistic disciplines, including food safety, public health, health economics, ecological health, social science, and animal health [141]. To manage food safety and comprehend the factors that contribute to the formation and persistence of hazards to people, animals, and the environment, one health is required [142].

Consistent surveillance for zoonotic illnesses should combine animal, human, and environmental markers, offering a useful tool for early detection of zoonotic infections [11]. Scientific assessment techniques, such as mathematical models, should first elucidate the interactions between animals, humans, and the environment before evaluating the impact of various policy alternatives [11]. Inadequate efforts have been made to prevent and manage zoonotic illnesses at their source, reflecting our incomplete knowledge of the underlying mechanisms of transmission in the animal reservoir. To effectively monitor and infer disease trends in animal reservoirs, present surveillance and model assessment should be upgraded [11]. It is crucial to approach them from a risk perspective in order to prioritise surveillance and interventions in the areas where the risks are greatest [143, 144]. In comparison to more stringent strategies like market shutdown, implementing the One Health strategy would be more sustainable in reducing the possibility of future zoonotic epidemics.

7.2 Biosecurity and biosafety strategies

In order to adequately analyse the zoonotic dangers, Naguib et al. [11] advocated a scientifically based risk-assessment framework that included field surveillance and risk assessment. In order to comprehend the real frequency of risks and the areas where the danger for disease onset is greatest, long-term, extensive surveillance is crucial. Along the value chains, food goods, the environment, customers, vendors, and vendors themselves would all be sampled and interviewed [11]. Rapid risk assessment seeks to investigate the environmental and zoonotic background, as well as the transmission potential of the present and upcoming zoonotic outbreaks, with the use of this all-encompassing surveillance system [11]. Emergency response in high-risk locations and routine treatments in low- to medium-risk areas would be used to leverage risk-based hierarchical controls [11].

7.3 Sustainable slaughterhouse and wet market management

Cross-species spread of infectious illnesses has been connected to inappropriate animal storage, crowding, poor hygiene, incorrect faeces disposal, and improper carcass disposal in wet markets [25]. Wet marketplaces that deal locally in cattle products have been made into epicentres of infectious diseases due to the lax implementation of food safety regulations. Aiyar and Pingali [25] define a wet market as an open food market. Traditionally, the primary qualities of wet market is a location that sells live animals in the open. Pigs, fish, reptiles, and poultry may be part of the collection of animals traded [33]. To reduce the risks to public health from endemic diseases as well as emerging diseases, markets must gradually improve with better food safety, hygiene standards, less animal crowding, and regular inspections from reputable officials with the authority to sample and condemn products [11].

7.4 Individualised animal treatment

The ideal course of action is to postpone and, avoid the appearance and subsequent spread of resistant bacteria or resistance genes, according to the case study of Antimicrobial Resistance (AMR). The widespread use of antimicrobial agents in veterinary medicine to treat both food animals and companion animals cannot be utilised to make up for substandard animal care and raising conditions [142]. Preventative medicine needs to be improved, including better biosecurity, reinforcement of animal health and welfare within production systems, improved access to infection-prevention vaccines, and an increase in animal breeding programmes that focus on robustness and resilience [142]. The creation of an efficient surveillance system, as well as extensive education and training of several system actors within the Animal Source Foods (ASF) system, are likely necessary to achieve sustainable antimicrobial usage.

7.5 Agricultural disease management synergy and policy monitoring activities

Integrating food safety objectives for disease prevention with trade-related food safety guidelines will support commerce and sustain competitiveness One such regulation that may be utilised to assist nations in achieving the twin objectives of equitable trade and improved health through food-safety investments is the Codex Alimentarius, an international convention for food safety [25]. Local stakeholders must be actively involved in the standards' implementation as well as active surveillance for containment to be successful [145]. Only if knowledge is shared transparently and local actors are given the means to address disease hazards can disease transmission be contained [25]. In the one-health, health, and food systems groups, improving interdepartmental collaboration can shorten the time it takes to identify diseases and execute containment measures [30, 146]. A "One Health" approach to food safety is one that aims to provide "optimal health for humans, animals, and the environment via the combined effort of different disciplines working locally, regionally, and internationally" [147]. If such an approach were used to address food safety, it might have the potential to combine the knowledge and resources from a variety of health domains, such as those in the fields of plant pathology, human and veterinary medicine, and ecology and wildlife and aquatic health [33]. By tracing and disrupting the pathways that lead to food contamination, these transdisciplinary synergies could provide crucial insights into the sources, reservoirs, and factors that underlie the emergence of infectious diseases and prevent the negative health effects associated with the emergence and spread of novel, emerging, or reemerging food-borne diseases [33].

Governments and funding organisations have moved quickly to support COVID-19-related research due to the race to understand the pathophysiology and epidemiology of the disease [148]. Such global finance and cooperation were not always obvious. SARS and H5N1 avian influenza, two foodborne zoonosis that first appeared in China, previously failed to garner the attention of the international community [41], limiting opportunities to improve disease surveillance systems that could provide risk assessments for the preparation and consumption of animal-sourced food [119]. Integrated animal, livestock, and human disease surveillance-response may help avoid future zoonoses outbreaks even if more research is needed to determine the zoonotic origin of COVID-19 [149]. Overall, consumers are becoming more aware of the wider public health implications of present food systems, despite the fact that there are still significant obstacles to overcome with regard to the reorientation of market incentives and food safety standards [72]. Future foodborne zoonoses treatments focused at informal markets may receive more support from national and international governments as a result of this increasing knowledge, which may improve policymakers' willingness to restructure global food systems to better safeguard public health [41]. As the incidence of events like foodborne zoonotic diseases and food safety are increasingly linked to globalised food systems, policymakers must focus on planning and prioritising response [139].

7.6 Food safety conservation measure

Experts in food safety should support research into preserving the genetic variety of cattle and other food production animals through creation of vaccines and veterinary services for livestock [25]. These measures can lessen the risk of escalating antimicrobial resistance as well as the vulnerability of animals to zoonotic infections [29, 150]. Increasing conservation activities will lessen exposure to animals that act as harmful disease vectors by reducing demand for wildlife and/or encouraging afforestation [28]. These initiatives will be critical to reducing the spread of zoonotic illnesses with a high risk but low likelihood [25].

7.7 Life Cycle Thinking (LCT)

A crucial idea in accomplishing the shift to a more ecologically sustainable food system is Life Cycle Thinking (LCT) [151]. Along the life cycle of complex food systems, it enables the evaluation of inputs, outputs, and potential environmental implications. LCT is defined as "moving beyond the conventional focus on production locations and manufacturing methods to encompass environmental, social, and economic aspects of a product across its whole life cycle" according to the UNEP/SETAC Life Cycle Initiative [152]. LCA is the most preferred and frequently used tool to evaluate and address the environmental sustainability of food systems when dealing with current global challenges, such as ensuring food safety and environmental sustainability of food systems under conditions of climate change [65]. The primary environmental loads may be identified via LCA, allowing for more effective definition and implementation of reform initiatives. LCA must switch from its global viewpoint to RA's narrow, site-specific focus. These days, site-dependent characterisation variables [153], national databases [154, 155], and grid cell-based inventories [156] can all be used to do. These Worldwide programmes and activities are driven by this global problem, which is already included in the portfolio of policy objectives [65].

8. Review of recent research of novel detection and control techniques in addressing the public health threat posed by foodborne zoonotic illness

Food safety laboratories can find new infections and detect pathogen deviations through routine testing, monitoring, and participation in epidemiological

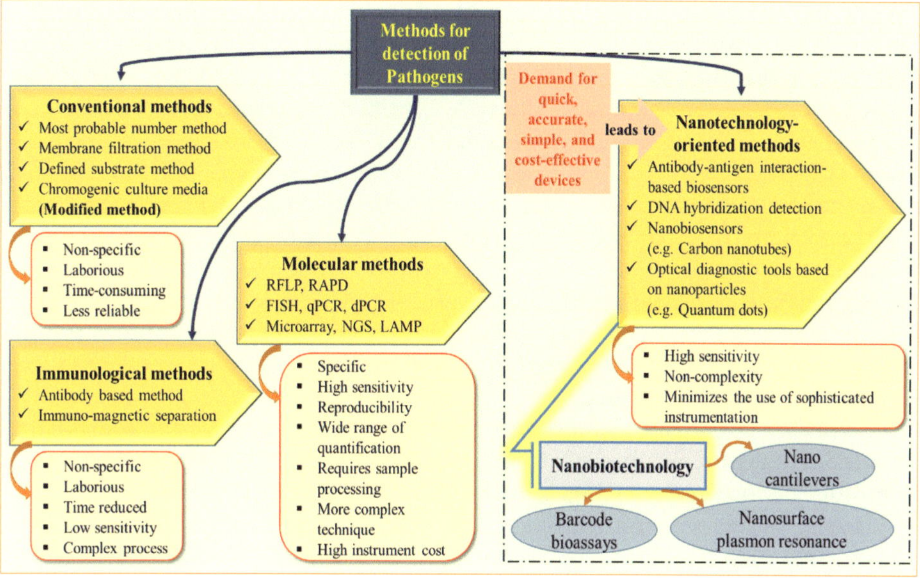

Figure 2.
Standard and novel techniques for the detection and control of foodborne zoonotic pathogens. Source: Shanker et al. [157], Sahoo et al. [139].

investigations. Controlling foodborne outbreaks requires quick identification of the infection pathway and focused detection of the causing organisms. The source may be looked into using the several detection techniques shown in **Figure 2** [139]. Bacteriophages, or "phages" for short, are a possible replacement for conventional methods of food safety preservation [82], particularly given their effectiveness against bacteria that are resistant to antibiotics [158]. Phage-based food treatments reduce the loads of spoilage microorganisms in fruits, dairy products, poultry, and red meats as well as dangerous bacteria such *L. monocytogenes, Salmonella*, and *C. jejuni* [159].

Molecular-based assays such as next-generation sequencing (NGS), quantitative and digital polymerase chain reaction (qPCR and dPCR), immunomagnetic separation assays, florescence in situ hybridization (FISH), DNA microarrays, direct epifluorescence filter techniques, latex agglutination tests, and flow cytometry are more sensitive than traditional culture methods for the rapid detection of pathogens [17]. Whole-genome sequencing (WGS), an analytical technique used to determine an organism's complete genomic sequence, foodborne pathogen routine monitoring and surveillance, tracing contamination sources, demarcating transmission routes in the farm-to-fork continuum, and incorporating genomic data into microbiological risk assessment, is a widely used application of NGS [160].

Cutting-edge genomic technologies are opening up fascinating new possibilities for zoonotic pathogen surveillance in a variety of contexts and ecosystems. Using taxonomically informative genes, such as the 16S rRNA gene, next-generation sequencing systems enable the metabarcoding of complex bacterial communities [161]. As a molecular marker for bacterial identification, including for pathogens with clinical significance, 16S rRNA sequence data are particularly helpful [162]. While second-generation sequencing platforms, such as Illumina MiSeq and NextSeq, which are frequently used for bacterial metabarcoding experiments, offer high per-base accuracy and sequencing throughput, the resulting data are only relatively short (300 bp) reads, which frequently allow for the analysis of specific subregions of the 16S rRNA gene's full-length (1550 bp) sequence [163].

The Oxford Nanopore Technologies (ONT) MinION sequencer, on the other hand, is a third-generation single-molecule sequencing device that can sequence unusually lengthy DNA fragments (i.e., hundreds to millions of bases in length) [164]. Because of this, the MinION can sequence the complete 16S rRNA gene, which has a length of 1550 base pairs, offering two to five times the coverage of the 16S rRNA gene compared to second-generation sequencing data. A higher number of phylogenetically relevant characteristics are included in full-length 16S sequencing data, which improves downstream bacterial taxonomy identification [161]. This strategy is crucial because, according to Byrd et al. [165], bacterial pathogenicity is often seen as a species- or strain-level phenomena.

On-site cost-effective quick analytical detection techniques are a new challenge compared to traditional approaches, claimed Sahoo et al. [139]. Potential exists for combining chemical engineering, biosensors, microfluids, and nanotechnology [166]. Large surface areas of nanomaterials make it possible for various biomolecules and reaction sites to engage with a target species [139]. This characteristic allows for the creation of sensitive nanobiosensors with faster reaction times for precise detection, in conjunction with the superior optical and electrical capabilities of nanomaterials [167]. In order to create a piezoelectric biosensor for "real-time" detection of the foodborne pathogen *E. coli* O157:H7, the electrical characteristics of the Au NPs were taken advantage of [168]. *E. coli* and *Campylobacter* have been removed from poultry products using nanoparticles [169]. Using magnetic nanoparticle-based immunomagnetic separation and real-time PCR, *Listeria monocytogenes* was found in milk samples [157]. For the quick detection of *Salmonella enteritidis*, two nanoparticle-based fluorescent barcoded DNA assays were developed. Using a portable device and a nanosensor, researchers found cytochrome b genes in animal diets [170].

9. Conclusions

The zoonotic spread of foodborne illness is presently a danger to the complex and dynamic global food system. Food losses and waste, a decline in optimal nutrition and dietary intake, and the effects of infectious diseases on human health on the production and distribution of food are all signs of their impact on global food safety and nutrition security. It is crucial to control foodborne zoonotic diseases using a variety of food system approaches, including Man-imal One Health Strategies, Biosecurity and Biosafety Strategies, Sustainable Slaughterhouse and Wet Market Management, Individualised Animal Treatment, Agricultural Disease Management Synergy and Policy Monitoring Activities, Food Safety Conservation Measure, and Life Cycle Thinking (LCT).

With the advancement of chemical engineering, biosensors, microfluids, and nanotechnology, more sensitive molecular-based assays for the rapid detection of pathogens have been developed. These include next-generation sequencing (NGS), quantitative and digital polymerase chain reaction (qPCR and dPCR), immunomagnetic separation assays, fluorescence in situ hybridization (FISH), DNA microarrays, direct epifluorescence filter techniques, latex agglutination tests, A collaborative, coordinated, multidisciplinary, responsible, cross-sectoral approach including ministries and institutions involved in commerce, health, and agriculture at regional, national, and international levels is needed for prompt identification and treatment to new infectious pathogens.

Conflict of interest

The authors declare no conflict of interest.

Author details

Elechi Jasper Okoro Godwin[1*], Vidhya Chandrasekaran[2], Adamu Cornelius Smah[3] and Ekoja Omeyi Faith[4]

1 Department of Pharmacy, Health and Nutritional Sciences, University of Calabria, Rende, CS, Italy

2 Department of Primary Processing Storage and Handling, National Institute of Food Technology, Entrepreneurship and Management, Thanjavur (NIFTEM-T), Tamil Nadu, India

3 Department of Public Health and Food Safety, École nationale vétérinaire, agroalimentaire et de l'alimentation de Nantes-Atlantique, Nantes, France

4 Faculty of Science and Technology, Department of Environmental Contamination and Toxicology, University of Bask Country, Spain

*Address all correspondence to: helloeljasper@gmail.com

IntechOpen

© 2022 The Author(s). Licensee IntechOpen. This chapter is distributed under the terms of the Creative Commons Attribution License (http://creativecommons.org/licenses/by/3.0), which permits unrestricted use, distribution, and reproduction in any medium, provided the original work is properly cited.

References

[1] FAO. Thinking About the Future of Food Safety—A Foresight Report. Rome; 2022. DOI: 10.4060/cb8667en

[2] Fanzo JC. Fixing Dinner Fix the Planet? Johns Hopkins University Press; 2021. DOI: 10.1353/book.83887

[3] Jones KE, Patel NG, Levy MA, Storeygard A, Balk D, Gittleman JL, et al. Global trends in emerging infectious diseases. Nature. 2008;**451**(7181):990-993

[4] Rohr JR, Barrett CB, Civitello DJ, Craft ME, Delius B, DeLeo GA, et al. Emerging human infectious diseases and the links to global food production. Nature Sustainability. 2019;**2**:445-456 10.1038/s41893-019-0293-3

[5] Roberts L. Nigeria's invisible crisis. Science. 2017;**356**:18-23

[6] Naylor R. The Evolving Sphere of Food Security. Oxford Univ. Press; 2014

[7] FAO and WHO. The Rome Declaration on Nutrition. Second International Conference on Nutrition. Rome: Food and Agriculture Organization of the United Nations; 2014

[8] United Nations. Transforming Our World: The 2030 Agenda for Sustainable Development (a/RES/70/1). New York, NY; 2015. https://sustainabledevelopment.un.org/content/documents/21252030%20Agenda%20for%20Sustainable%20Development%20web.pdf

[9] FAO. Climate change: Unpacking the burden on food safety. Food Safety and Quality Series. 2020;**8**:176 https://www.fao.org/documents/card/en/c/ca8185en/

[10] UNEP and ILRI. Preventing the Next Pandemic: Zoonotic Diseases and How to Break the Chain of Transmission. Nairobi, Kenya: United Nations Environment Programme and International Livestock Research Institute; 2020

[11] Naguib MM, Li R, Ling J, Grace D, Nguyen-Viet H, Johanna F. Lindahl live and wet markets: Food access versus the risk of disease emergence. Trends in Microbiology. 2021;**29**(7). DOI: 10.1016/j.tim.2021.02.007

[12] Kruse H, Kirkemo A-M, Handeland K. Wildlife as source of zoonotic infections. Emerging Infectious Diseases. 2004;**10**(12):2067-2072

[13] Webster RG. Wet markets—A continuing source of severe acute respiratory syndrome and influenza? Lancet. 2004;**363**:234-236

[14] EFSA European Food Safety Authority. The European Union one health 2020 zoonoses report European Centre for disease prevention and control. EFSA Journal. 2021;**19**(12):6971 https://efsa.onlinelibrary.wiley.com/doi/epdf/10.2903/j.efsa.2021.6971

[15] Brucellosis PM. A highly infectious foodborne zoonotic disease of public health concern Madridge. Journal of Food Science and Technology. 2018;**S1**(1):1-3. DOI: 10.18689/mjft-2577-4182-S1-101

[16] Abebe E, Gugsa G, Ahmed M. Review on major food-borne zoonotic bacterial pathogens. Journal of Tropical Medicine. 2020. DOI: 10.1155/2020/4674235

[17] Dhama KS, Rajagunalan SC, et al. Food-borne pathogens of animal

origin-diagnosis, prevention, control and their zoonotic significance: A review. Pakistan Journal of Biological Sciences. 2013;**16**(20):1076-1085

[18] Addis M, Sisay D. A review on major food borne bacterial illnesses. Journal of Tropical Diseases. 2015;**3**(4):1-7

[19] Chlebicz A, Śliżewska K. Campylobacteriosis, salmonellosis, yersiniosis, and listeriosis as zoonotic foodborne diseases: A review. International Journal of Environmental Research and Public Health. 2018;**15**(5):1-28

[20] Bidaisee S, Macpherson CNL. Zoonoses and one health: A review of the literature. Journal of Parasitology. 2014;**2014**

[21] Carrique-Mas JJ, Bryant J. A review of foodborne bacterial and parasitic zoonoses in Vietnam. EcoHealth. 2013;**10**(4):465-489

[22] Abunna F, Abriham T, Gizaw F, et al. Staphylococcus: Isolation, identification and antimicrobial resistance in dairy cattle farms, municipal abattoir and personnel in and around Asella, Ethiopia. Journal of Veterinary Science & Technology. 2016;7(6):1-7

[23] Hemalata VB, Virupakshaiah DBM. Isolation and identification of food borne pathogens from spoiled food samples. International Journal of Current Microbiology and Applied Sciences. 2016;**5**(6):1017-1025

[24] Argaw S, Addis M. A review on staphylococcal food poisoning. Food Science and Quality Management. 2015;**40**:59-71

[25] Aiyar A, Pingali P. Pandemics and food systems-towards a proactive food safety approach to disease prevention & management. Food Security. 2020;**12**(4):749-756. DOI: 10.1007/s12571-020-01074-3

[26] Destoumieux-Garzón D, Mavingui P, Boëtsch G, Boissier J, Darriet F, Duboz P, et al. The one health concept: 10 years old and a long road ahead. Frontiers in Veterinary Science. 2018;**5**(14)

[27] Han BA, Kramer AM, Drake JM. Global patterns of zoonotic disease in mammals. Trends in Parasitology. 2016;**32**(7):565-577. DOI: 10.1016/j.pt.2016.04.007

[28] Hassell JM, Begon M, Ward MJ, Fèvre EM. Urbanization and disease emergence: Dynamics at the wildlife—Live-stock—Human Interface. Trends in Ecology & Evolution. 2017;**32**(1):55-67. DOI: 10.1016/j.tree.2016.09.012

[29] Holmes AH, Moore LSP, Sundsfjord A, Steinbakk M, Regmi S, Karkey A, et al. Understanding the mechanisms and drivers of antimicrobial resistance. The Lancet. 2016;**387**(10014):176-187. DOI: 10.1016/S0140-6736(15)00473-0

[30] Morse SS, Mazet JAK, Woolhouse M, Parrish CR, Carroll D, Karesh WB, et al. Prediction and prevention of the next pandemic zoonosis. The Lancet. 2012;**380**(9857):1956-1965. DOI: 10.1016/S0140-6736(12)61684-5

[31] King L. What is One Health and Why Is It Relevant to Food Safety? Presentation Given at the, Public Workshop Improving Food Safety Through One Health, Forum on Microbial Threats. Washington, DC: Institute of Medicine; 2011

[32] IOM (Institute of Medicine). Microbial Threats to Health: Emergence, Detection, and Response. Washington, DC: The National Academies Press; 2003

[33] Choffnes Eileen R, Relman DA, Olsen LA, Hutton R, Mack A. Improving Food Safety Through a One Health Approach: Workshop Summary. Rapporteurs; Forum on Microbial Threats; Board on Global Health. Washington, DC: Institute of Medicine; 2012 Available from The National Academies Press at http://www.nap.edu/catalog.php?record_id=13423

[34] IOM (Institute of Medicine). Emerging Infections: Microbial Threats to Health in the United States. Washington, DC: National Academy Press; 1992

[35] IOM (Institute of Medicine) and NRC (National Research Council). Sustaining Global Surveillance and Response to Emerging Zoonotic Diseases. Washington, DC: The National Academies Press; 2009

[36] King LJ. Emerging zoonoes and pathogens of public health concern. Revue Scientifique et Technique de l'OIE. 2004;**23**(2):429-433

[37] Pike BL, Saylors KE, Fair JN, LeBreton M, Tamoufe U, Djoko CF, et al. The origination and prevention of pandemics. Emerging Infections. 2010;**50**(12):1636-1640

[38] Rasko DA, Webster DR, Sahl JW, Bashir A, Boisen N, Scheutz F, et al. Origins of the *E. coli* strain causing an outbreak of hemolytic-uremic syndrome in Germany. New England Journal of Medicine. 2011;**365**(8):709-717

[39] Abebe E, Gugsa G, Ahmed M. Review on major food-borne zoonotic bacterial pathogens. Journal of Tropical Medicine. 2020;**2020**

[40] Taylor LH, Latham SM, Woolhouse MEJ. Risk factors for human disease emergence. Philosophical Transactions of the Royal Society of London B. 2001;**356**:983-989

[41] GAIN (Global Alliance for Improved Nutrition). Assessing Food Safety Interventions Relevant to Foodborne Zoonoses in Low- and Middle-Income Countries. A USAID EatSafe Project Report 2020

[42] Shi M et al. The evolutionary history of vertebrate RNA viruses. Nature. 2018;**556**:197-202

[43] Shi M et al. Redefining the invertebrate RNA virosphere. Nature. 2016;**540**:539-543

[44] Heredia N, Santos G. Animals as sources of food-borne pathogens: A review. Animal. Nutrition. 2018;**4**:250-255. DOI: 10.1016/j.aninu.2018.04.006

[45] Kaakoush NO, Casta~no-Rodríguez N, Mitchell HM, Mana SM. Global epidemiology of Campylobacter infection. Clinical Microbiology Reviews. 2015;**28**:687-720

[46] EFSA. Scientific opinion on quantification of the risk posed by broiler meat to human campylobacteriosis in the EU. EFSA Journal. 2010;**8**:1437-1526

[47] Silva J, Leite D, Fernandes M, Mena C, Gibb PA, Teixeira P. Campylobacter spp. as a foodborne pathogen: A review. Frontiers in Microbiology. 2011;**2**:1-12

[48] Buchanan RL, Gorris LGM, Hayman MM, Jackson TC, Whiting RC. A review of *Listeria monocytogenes*: An update on outbreaks, virulence, dose-response, ecology, and risk assessments. Food Control. 2017;**75**:1-13

[49] Tilman D, Cassman KG, Matson PA, Naylor R, Polasky S. Agricultural

sustainability and intensive production practices. Nature. 2002;**418**:671-677

[50] United Nations, World Population Prospects: 2017. Revision: http://esa.un.org/unpd/wpp/

[51] Foley JA et al. Solutions for a cultivated planet. Nature. 2011;**478**:337-342

[52] Elechi JOG, Nwiyi IU, Adamu CS. Global food system transformation for resilience. In: Ribeiro-Barros AI, Tevera D, Goulao LF, Tivana LD, editors. Food Systems Resilience. London, UK: IntechOpen Limited; 2022. DOI: 10.5772/intechopen.102749

[53] Godfray HCJ, Garnett T. Food security and sustainable intensification. Philosophical Transactions of the Royal Society of London B. 2014;**369**:20120273

[54] FAO. How to Feed the World: Global Agriculture Towards 2050. FAO; 2009 www.fao.org/fileadmin/templates/wsfs/docs/Issues_papers/HLEF2050_Global_Agriculture.pdf

[55] FAO. World Agriculture Towards 2030/2050: 2012 Revision ESA Working Paper. FAO; 2012

[56] Lozano R et al. Global and regional mortality from 235 causes of death for 20 age groups in 1990 and 2010: A systematic analysis for the global burden of disease study. 2010. The Lancet. 2013;**380**:2095-2128

[57] Sheahan M, Barrett CB, Goldvale C. Human health and pesticide use in sub-Saharan Africa. Agricultural Economics. 2017;**48**:27-41

[58] Dobson A, Foufopoulos J. Emerging infectious pathogens of wildlife. Philosophical Transactions of the Royal Society of London B. 2001;**356**:1001-1012

[59] Evenson RE, Gollin D. Assessing the impact of the green revolution, 1960 to 2000. Science. 2003;**300**:758-762

[60] Mario H, Mason-D'Croz D, Thornton PK, Fanzo J, Rushton J, Godde C, et al. Livestock and sustainable food systems: status, trends, and priority actions. In: Food Systems Summit Brief. United Nations Food Systems Summit 2021. Scientific Group; 2021. https://sc-fss2021.org/

[61] Pingali P. Westernization of Asian diets and the transformationof food systems: Implications for research and policy. Food Policy. 2007;**32**(3):281-298. DOI: 10.1016/j.foodpol.2006.08.001

[62] Duffy M. Economies of size in production agriculture. Journal of Hunger & Environmental Nutrition. 2009;**4**(3-4):375-392

[63] Gorbach SL. Antimicrobial use in animal feed—Time to stop. The New England Journal of Medicine. 2001;**345**:1202-1203

[64] Van Boeckel TP et al. Reducing antimicrobial use in food animals. Science. 2017;**357**:1350-1352

[65] Feliciano RJ, Guzm'an-Luna P, Bou'e G, Mauricio-Iglesias M, Hospido A, Membr'e J-M. Strategies to mitigate food safety risk while minimizing environmental impacts in the era of climate change. Trends in Food Science & Technology. 2022. DOI: 10.1016/j.tifs.2022.02.027

[66] WHO. Food Safety, Climate Change and the Role of WHO. 2019. https://www.who.int/publications/i/item/food-safety-climate-change-and-the-role-of-who

[67] IPCC. In: Pachauri RK, Meyer LA, editors. Climate Change 2014: Synthesis Report. Contribution

of Working Groups I, II and III to the Fifth Assessment Report of the Intergovernmental Panel on Climate Change (Core Writing Team). 2015. https://www.ipcc.ch/report/ar5/syr/

[68] Jones BA, Grace D, Kock R, Alonso S, Rushton J, Said MY, et al. Zoonosis emergence linked to agricultural intensification and environmental change. Proceedings of the National Academy of Sciences. 2013;**110**(21):8399-8404

[69] Gould EA, Higgs S. Impact of climate change and other factors on emerging arbovirus diseases. Transactions of the Royal Society of Tropical Medicine and Hygiene. 2009;**103**(2):109-121. DOI: 10.1016/j.trstmh.2008.07.025

[70] Grace D, Mahuku G, Hoffmann V, Atherstone C, et al. International agricultural research to reduce food risks: Case studies on aflatoxins. Food Security. 2015;**7**(3):569-582. DOI: 10.1007/s12571-015-0469-2

[71] Li A, Kroeze C, Kahil T, Ma L, Strokal M. Water pollution from food production: Lessons for optimistic and optimal solutions. Current Opinion in Environmental Sustainability. 2019;**40**:88-94. DOI: 10.1016/j.cosust.2019.09.007

[72] Thomas LF, Patterson G, Coyne L, Rushton J. Countering the double-whammy of zoonotic diseases. Rural 21. 2020

[73] Béné C. Resilience of local food systems and links to food security—A review of some important concepts in the context of COVID-19 and other shocks. Food Security. 2020:1-18

[74] Hafez HM, Attia YA. Challenges to the poultry industry: Current perspectives and strategic future after the COVID-19 outbreak. Frontiers in Veterinary Science. 2020;**7**:516. DOI: 10.3389/fvets.2020.00516

[75] Kirk MD, Pires SM, Black RE, Caipo M, Crump JA, Devleesschauwer B, et al. World Health Organization estimates of the global and regional disease burden of 22 foodborne bacterial, protozoal, and viral diseases, 2010: A data synthesis. PLoS Medicine. 2015;**12**:e1001921

[76] Sharafutdinov I, Tegtmeyer N, Müsken M, Backert S. *Campylobacter jejuni* serine protease HtrA induces paracellular transmigration of microbiota across polarized intestinal epithelial cells. Biomolecules. 2022;**12**:521. DOI: 10.3390/biom12040521

[77] Burnham PM, Hendrixson DR. *Campylobacter jejuni*: Collective components promoting a successful enteric lifestyle. Nature Reviews Microbiology. 2018;**16**:551-565

[78] Heimesaat MM, Backert S, Alter T, Bereswill S. Human campylobacteriosis-a serious infectious threat in a one health perspective. Current Topics in Microbiology and Immunology. 2021;**431**:1-23

[79] European Food Safety Authority (EFSA). The European Union summary report on trends and sources of zoonoses, zoonotic agents and food-borne outbreaks in 2017. EFSA Journal. 2018;**16**:5500

[80] Center for Disease Control and Prevention (CDC). National Enteric Disease Surveillance: Salmonella Annual Summary. 2019. https://www.cdc.gov/nationalsurveillance/salmonella-surveillance.html

[81] Mezal EH, Sabol A, Khan MA, Ali N, Stefanova R, Khan AA. Isolation

and molecular characterization of Salmonella entericaserovar enteritidis from poultry house and clinical samples during 2010. Food Microbiology. 2014;**38**:67-74

[82] Rivera D, Moreno-Switt AI, Denes TG, Hudson LK, Peters TL, Samir R, et al. Novel Salmonella phage, vB_Sen_STGO-35-1, characterization and evaluation in chicken meat. Microorganisms. 2022;**10**:606. DOI: 10.3390/microorganisms10030606

[83] Majowicz SE, Musto J, Scallan E, Angulo FJ, Kirk M, O'Brien SJ, et al. The global burden of nontyphoidal Salmonella gastroenteritis. Clinical Infectious Diseases. 2010;**50**:882-889

[84] Jemmi T, Stephan R. *Listeria monocytogenes*: Food-borne pathogen and hygiene indicator. Revue Scientifique et Technique de l'OIE. 2006;**25**(2):571-580

[85] Scallan E, Hoekstra RM, Angulo FJ, Tauxe RV, Widdowson MA, Roy SL, et al. Foodborne illness acquired in the United States—Major pathogens. Emerging Infectious Diseases. 2011;**17**(1):7-15

[86] South Africa, National Institute for Communicable Diseases [SANICD]. An Update on the Outbreak of *Listeria monocytogenes*. South Africa: NICD; 2019 http://www.nicd.ac.za/wp-content/uploads/2018/08/An-update-on-the-outbreak-of-Listeria-monocytogenes-South-Africa.pdf

[87] Ghandhi M, Chikindas ML. Listeria: A foodborne pathogen that knows how to survive. International Journal of Food Microbiology. 2007;**113**:1-15

[88] Garcia A, Fox JG, Besser TE. Zoonotic enterohemorrhagic *Eschericia coli*: A one health perspective. ILAR Journal. 2010;**51**(3):221-232

[89] CDC (Centers for Disease Control and Prevention). 2011. FoodNet—Foodborne Diseases Active Surveillance Network. http://www.cdc.gov/foodnet/. [Accessed: January 23, 2012]

[90] Dean AS, Crump L, Greter H, Schelling E, Zinsstag J. Global burden of human brucellosis: A systematic review of disease frequency. PLoS Neglected Tropical Diseases. 2012;**6**(10):e1865

[91] Holubová N, Zikmundová V, Limpouchová Z, Sak B, KonečnýR. and Hlásková L. *Cryptosporidium proventriculisp*. n. (Apicomplexa: Cryptosporidiidae) in Psittaciformes birds. European Journal of Protistology. 2019;**69**:70-87

[92] Müller B, Dürr S, Alonso S, Hattendorf J, Laisse CJ, Parsons SD, et al. Zoonotic Mycobacterium bovis–induced tuberculosis in humans. Emerging Infectious Diseases. 2013;**19**(6):899

[93] Li M, Havelaar AH, Hoffmann S, Hald T, Kirk MD, Torgerson PR, et al. Global disease burden of pathogens in animal source foods, 2010. PLoS One. 2019;**14**(6):e0216545

[94] Yoshida A, Doanh PN, Maruyama H. Paragonimus and paragonimiasis in Asia: an update. Acta Tropica. 2019;**199**:105074

[95] Foreyt WJ, Abbott RC, Van Riper C. Trichinosis. Circular. 2013

[96] Rostami A, Gamble HR, Dupouy-Camet J, Khazan H, Bruschi F. Meat sources of infection for outbreaks of human trichinellosis. Food Microbiology. 2017;**64**:65-71

[97] Pavel R, Ursoniu S, Paduraru AA, Lighezan R, Lupu MA, Olariu TR. Seroprevalence and risk factors of trichinella spiralis infection in blood donors from Western Romania.

Medicina. 2022;**58**:128. DOI: 10.3390/medicina58010128

[98] Hoofnagle JH, Nelson KE, Purcell RH. Hepatitis E. The New England Journal of Medicine. 2012;**367**(13):1237-1244

[99] Meng XJ. Hepatitis E virus: Animal reservoirs and zoonotic risk. Veterinary Microbiology. 2010;**140**(3-4):256-265

[100] Meng XJ. From barnyard to food table: The omnipresence of hepatitis E virus and risk for zoonotic infection and food safety. Virus Research. 2011;**161**(1):23-30

[101] Treagus S, Wright C, Baker-Austin C, et al. The foodborne transmission of hepatitis E virus to humans. Food and Environmental Virology. 2021;**13**:127-145. DOI: 10.1007/s12560-021-09461-5

[102] Rein DB, Stevens GA, Theaker J, Wittenborn JS, Wiersma ST. The global burden of hepatitis E virus genotypes 1 and 2 in 2005. Hepatology. 2012;**55**(4):988-997

[103] WHO. Monkeypox. 2022. https://www.who.int/news-room/fact-sheets/detail/monkeypox

[104] Halpin K, Hyatt AD, Fogarty R, Middleton D, Bingham J, Epstein JH, et al. Pteropid bats are confirmed as the reservoir hosts of henipaviruses: A comprehensive experimental study of virus transmission. American Journal of Tropical Medicine and Hygiene. 2011;**85**:946-951

[105] Luby SP, Gurley ES, Hossain MJ. Transmission of human infection with Nipah virus. Clinical Infectious Diseases. 2009;**49**(11):1743-1748

[106] Epstein JH, Field HE, Luby S, Pulliam JR, Daszak P. Nipah virus: Impact, origins, and causes of emergence. Current Infectious Disease Reports. 2006;**8**(1):59-65

[107] Libera K, Konieczny K, Grabska J, Szopka W, Augustyniak A, Pomorska-Mól M. Selected livestock-associated zoonoses as a growing challenge for public health. Infectious Disease Reports. 2022;**14**:63-81. DOI: 10.3390/idr14010008

[108] FAO. World Food and Agriculture—Statistical Yearbook 2021. Rome, Italy: FAO; 2021

[109] Zhou X, Wang Y, Liu H, Guo F, Doi SA, Smith C, et al. Effectiveness of market-level biosecurity at reducing exposure of poultry and humans to avian influenza: A systematic review and meta-analysis. The Journal of Infectious Diseases. 2018;**218**:1861-1875

[110] Turlewicz-Podbielska H, Pomorska-Mól M. Swine diseases caused by circoviruses and swine influenza according to data from the 11th European symposium of porcine health management (ESPHM) in Utrecht. Życie Weterynaryjne. 2019;**94**:804-809

[111] Li S, He Y, Mann DA, Deng X. Global spread of Salmonella enteritidis via centralized sourcing and international trade of poultry breeding stocks. Nature Communications. 2021;**12**:5109

[112] Tang JW, Shetty N, Lam TT-Y. Features of the new pandemic influenza a/H1N1/2009 virus: Virology, epidemiology, clinical and public health aspects. Current Opinion in Pulmonary Medicine. 2010;**16**:235-241

[113] Hilgenfeld R, Peiris M. From SARS to MERS: 10 years of research on highly pathogenic human coronaviruses.

Antiviral Research. 2013;**100**(1):286-295. DOI: 10.1016/j.antiviral.2013.08.015

[114] Knipe DM, Howley PM, Griffin D, Lamb R, Martin M. Filoviridae: Marburg and Ebola viruses. In: Fields Virology. 5th ed. Philadelphia, PA, USA: Lippincott Williams & Wilkins; 2006. pp. 1410-1448

[115] Ghareeb OA. Ebola—A fatal emerging zoonotic disease: A review. Annals of R.S.C.B. 2021;**25**(6):8748-8754

[116] Malvy D, McElroy AK, de Clerck H, Günther S, van Griensven J. Ebola virus disease. The Lancet. 2019;**393**(10174):936-948

[117] Leendertz SAJ, Gogarten JF, Düx A, Calvignac-Spencer S, Leendertz FH. Assessing the evidence supporting fruit bats as the primary reservoirs for Ebola viruses. EcoHealth. 2016;**13**(1):18-25. DOI: 10.1007/s10393-015-1053-0

[118] WHO. Introduction to Lassa Fever Managing Infectious Hazards. 2018. https://cdn.who.int/media/docs/default-source/documents/emergencies/health-topics---lassa-fever/lassa-fever-introduction.pdf?sfvrsn=b1b96509_2&download=true

[119] Shao D, Shi Z, Wei J, Ma Z. A brief review of foodborne zoonoses in China. Epidemiology & Infection. 2011;**139**(10):1497-1504

[120] Roe D, Dickman A, Kock R, Milner-Gulland E, Rihoy E. Beyond banning wildlife trade: COVID-19, conservation and development. World Development. 2020;**136**:105121

[121] FAO. (2019). The State of Food and Agriculture 2019: Moving Forward on Food Loss and Waste Reduction. http://www.fao.org/3/ca6030en/ca6030en.pdf. [Accessed: February 9, 2022]

[122] UNEP. Food Waste Index Report 2021. In United nations Environment Programme; 2021 https://www.unep.org/resources/report/unep-food-waste-index-report-2021

[123] Gauthier-Clerc M, Lebarbenchon C, Thomas F. Recent expansion of highly pathogenic avian influenza H5N1: A critical review. Ibis. 2007;**149**(2):202-214

[124] Burgos S, Burgos SA. Avian influenza outbreaks in Southeast Asia affects prices, markets and trade: A short case study. International Journal of Poultry Science. 2007;**6**(12):1006-1009

[125] Civitello DJ, Allman BE, Morozumi C, Rohr JR. Assessing the direct and indirect effects of food provisioning and nutrient enrichment on wildlife infectious disease dynamics. Philosophical Transactions of the Royal Society of London B. 2018;**373**:20170101

[126] Gross R, Schoeneberger H, Pfeifer H, Preuss HA. The Four Dimensions of Food and Nutrition Security: Definitions and Concepts. Rome, Italy: Food and Agriculture Organization of the United Nations; 2000

[127] ILRI. Project Brief: Participatory Risk Assessment of Pork in ha Noi and ha Tay, Vietnam. Improving the Competitiveness of Pig Producers in Vietnam Project Brief 3. Nairobi, Kenya: International Livestock Research Institute; 2010

[128] Cornelsen L, Alarcon P, Häsler B, Amendah DD, Ferguson E, Fevre EM, et al. Cross-sectional study of price and other drivers of demand for animal source foods in low-income urban areas of Nairobi, Kenya. BMC Nutrition. 2016;**2**:70. DOI: 10.1186/s40795-016-0109-z

[129] Grace D. Food safety in low- and middle-income countries. International Journal of Environmental Research and Public Health. 2015;**12**(9):10490-10507

[130] Barbara H, Dominguez-Salas P, Fornace K, Garza M, Grace D, Rushton J. Where food safety meets nutrition outcomes in livestock and fish value chains: A conceptual approach. Food Security. 2017. DOI: 10.1007/s12571-017-0710-2

[131] Kavle JA, El-Zanaty F, Landry M, Galloway R. The rise in stunting in relation to avian influenza and food consumption patterns in Lower Egypt in comparison to upper Egypt: Results from 2005 and 2008 demographic and health surveys. BMC Public Health. 2015;**15**. DOI: 10.1186/s12889-015-1627-3

[132] Knutie SA, Wilkinson CL, Wu QC, Ortega CN, Rohr JR. Host resistance and tolerance of parasitic gut worms depend on resource availability. Oecologia. 2017;**183**:1031-1040

[133] Young SL, Sherman PW, Lucks JB, Pelto GH. Why on earth? Evaluating hypotheses about the physiological functions of human geophagy. The Quarterly Review of Biology. 2011;**86**:97-120

[134] Pieracci GE, Hall JA, Gharpure R, Haile A, Walelign E, Deressa A, et al. Prioritizing zoonotic diseases in Ethiopia using a one health approach. One Health. 2016;**2**:131-135. DOI: 10.1016/j.onehlt.2016.09.001PMID:28220151

[135] Grace D, Gilbert J, Randolph T, Kang'ethe E. The multiple burdens of zoonotic disease and an eco-health approach to their assessment. Tropical Animal Health and Production. 2012;**44**:67-73. DOI: 10.1007/s11250-012-0209-y PMID: 22886445

[136] Alsan M. The effect of the tsetse fly on African development. The American Economic Review. 2015;**105**:382-410

[137] Ngonghala CN et al. General ecological models for human subsistence, health and poverty. Nature Ecology & Evolution. 2017;**1**:1153-1159

[138] Barrett CB, Carter MR, Chavas J. The Economics of Poverty Traps. Univ. Chicago Press; 2019

[139] Monalisa S, Panigrahi C, Aradwad P. Management strategies emphasizing advanced food processing approaches to mitigate food borne zoonotic pathogens in food system. Food Frontiers. 2022:1-25. DOI: 10.1002/fft2.153

[140] FAO–OIE–WHO Collaboration. Sharing responsibilities and coordinating global activities to address health risks at the animal–human–ecosystems interfaces. A tripartite concept note. 2010. http://www.who.int/foodsafety/zoonoses/final_concept_note_Hanoi.pdf.

[141] Xie T, Liu W, Anderson BD, Liu X, Gray GC. A system dynamics approach to understanding the one health concept. PLoS One. 2017;**12**:e0184430

[142] Sofia B, Söderqvist K, Vågsholm I. Food safety challenges and one health within Europe. Acta Veterinaria Scandinavica. 2018;**60**:1. DOI: 10.1186/s13028-017-0355-3

[143] Grace D et al. Safe food, fair food: Participatory risk analysis for improving the safety of informally produced and marketed food in sub-Saharan Africa. Revue Africaine de Santé et de Productions Animales. 2010;**8**:3-11

[144] Roesel K, Grace D. Food Safety and Informal Markets: Animal Products in Sub-Saharan Africa. 1st ed. Routledge; 2014

[145] Häsler B, Gilbert W, Jones BA, Pfeiffer DU, Rushton J, Otte MJ. The economic value of one health in relation to the mitigation of zoonotic disease risks BT. In: Mackenzie JS, Jeggo M, Daszak P, Richt JA, editors. One Health: The Human-Animal-Environment Interfaces in Emerging Infectious Diseases: The Concept and Examples of a One Health Approach. Berlin Heidelberg: Springer; 2013. pp. 127-151. DOI: 10.1007/82_2012_239

[146] Kelly TR, Karesh WB, Johnson CK, Gilardi KVK, Anthony SJ, Goldstein T, et al. One health proof of concept: Bringing a transdisciplinary approach to surveillance for zoonotic viruses at the human-wild animal interface. Preventive Veterinary Medicine. 2017;**137**:112-118

[147] American Veterinary Medical Association AVMA. One health: A new professional imperative. One Health Initiative Task Force: Final Report. 2008;**2008**. https://www.avma.org/sites/default/files/resources/onehealth_final.pdf

[148] Prudêncio M, Costa JC. Research funding after COVID-19. Nature Microbiology. 2020;**5**(8):986

[149] Zinsstag J, Utzinger J, Probst-Hensch N, Shan L, Zhou X-N. Towards integrated surveillance-response systems for the prevention of future pandemics. Infectious Diseases of Poverty. 2020;**9**(1):1-6

[150] Marshall BM, Levy SB. Food animals and antimicrobials: Impacts on human health. Clinical Microbiology Reviews. 2011;**24**(4):718-733

[151] Notarnicola B, Sala S, Anton A, McLaren SJ, Saouter E, Sonesson U. The role of life cycle assessment in supporting sustainable agri-food systems: A review of the challenges. Journal of Cleaner Production. 2017;**140**:399-409. DOI: 10.1016/j.jclepro.2016.06.071

[152] Cycle Initiative L. What is Life Cycle Thinking?. 2016. https://www.lifecycleinitiative.org/starting-life-cycle-thinking/what-is-life-cycle-thinking/. [Accessed: January 20, 2021].

[153] Saouter E, Aschberger K, Fantke P, Hauschild MZ, Kienzler A, Paini A, et al. Improving substance information in USEtox®, part 2: Data for estimating fate and ecosystem exposure factors. Environmental Toxicology & Chemistry. 2017;**36**(12):3463-3470. DOI: 10.1002/etc.3903

[154] Environmental Protection Agency. 2017 National Emissions Inventory (NEI) Data Air Emissions Inventories. 2021. https://www.epa.gov/air-emissions-inventories/2017-national-emissions-inventory-nei-data

[155] NREL. U.S. Life Cycle Inventory Database. 2012. https://www.lcacommons.gov/nrel/search. [Accessed: January 20, 2021]

[156] Thakrar SK, Goodkind AL, Tessum CW, Marshall JD, Hill JD. Life cycle air quality impacts on human health from potential switchgrass production in the United States. Biomass and Bioenergy. 2018;**114**(June 2016):73-82. DOI: 10.1016/j.biombioe.2017.10.031

[157] Shanker R, Singh G, Jyoti A, Dwivedi PD, Singh SP. Nanotechnology and detection of microbial pathogens. In: Animal Biotechnology. Academic Press; 2020. pp. 593-611

[158] Kazi M, Annapure US. Bacteriophage biocontrol of foodborne pathogens. Journal of Food Science and Technology. 2016;**53**:1355-1362

[159] Rivera H, Hamilton-West D, Moreno-Switt P. Two Phages of the

genera Felixounavirus subjected to 12 hour challenge on Salmonella Infantis showed. Distinct Genotypic and Phenotypic Changes. Viruses. 2019;**11**:586

[160] EFSA and ECDC. The European Union summary report on trends and sources of zoonoses, zoonotic agents and food-borne outbreaks in 2015. EFSA Journal. 2016;**14**(12):4634. DOI: 10.2903/j.efsa.2016.4634

[161] Jahan NA, Lindsey LL, Kipp EJ, Reinschmidt A, Heins BJ, Runck AM, et al. Nanopore-based surveillance of zoonotic bacterial pathogens in farm-dwelling Peridomestic rodents. Pathogens. 2021;**10**:1183. DOI: 10.3390/pathogens10091183

[162] Sheahan T, Hakstol R, Kailasam S, Glaister GD, Hudson AJ, Wieden H-J. Rapid metagenomics analysis of EMS vehicles for monitoring pathogen load using nanopore DNA sequencing. PLoS One. 2019;**14**:e0219961

[163] Goodwin S, McPherson JD, McCombie WR. Coming of age: Ten years of next-generation sequencing technologies. Nature Reviews Genetics. 2016;**17**:333

[164] Tyler AD, Mataseje L, Urfano CJ, Schmidt L, Antonation KS, Mulvey MR, et al. Evaluation of Oxford Nanopore's MinION sequencing device for microbial whole genome sequencing applications. Scientific Reports. 2018;**8**:123

[165] Byrd AL, Belkaid Y, Segre JA. The human skin microbiome. Nature Reviews. Microbiology. 2018;**16**:143

[166] Azinheiro S, Kant K, Shahbazi M-A, Garrido-Maestu A, Prado M, Dieguez L. A smart microfluidic platform for rapid multiplexed detection of foodborne pathogens. Food Control. 2020;**114**:107242. DOI: 10.1016/j.foodcont.2020.107242

[167] Sahoo M, Vishwakarma S, Panigrahi C, Kumar J. Nanotechnology: Current applications and future scope in food. Food Frontiers. 2021;**2**(1):3-22

[168] Gilmartin N, O'Kennedy R. Nanobiotechnologies for the detection and reduction of pathogens. Enzyme and Microbial Technology. 2012;**50**(2):87-95

[169] Manuja A, Kumar B, Singh RK. Nanotechnology developments: Opportunities for animal health and production. Nanotechnology Development. 2012;**2**:e4. DOI: 10.4081/nd.2012.e4

[170] Zhang D, Carr DJ, Alocilja EC. Fluorescent bio-barcode DNA assay for the detection of *Salmonella enterica serovar enteritidis*. Biosensors and Bioelectronics. 2009;**24**(5):1377-1381

Chapter 3

Pathogenicity, Toxin Production, Control and Detection of *Bacillus cereus*

Barakatullah Mohammadi, Natasha Gorkina and Stephanie A. Smith

Abstract

Bacillus cereus is a toxin-producing, endospore-forming, facultative bacterium ubiquitous in the environment. It has been associated with numerous foodborne illness outbreaks and is found in a variety of foods including grains, produce and processed foods. When present in high numbers, *B. cereus* produces toxins leading to foodborne illness. Although disease is usually self-limiting and resolves with a short time, illness can result in complications. Moreover, *B. cereus* is resistant to many antimicrobials which can make treatment difficult in scenarios where more extensive treatment is required. Current control methods are limited, and detection of this pathogen in food is often difficult due to its genetic similarity to *Bacillus anthracis* and *Bacillus thuringiensis*. Given this, more research is required to identify better process controls to reduce contamination of food with this ubiquitous organism, and develop better methods for detection.

Keywords: *Bacillus cereus*, antimicrobial resistance, Bacillus, foodborne illness, detection, control, enterotoxins, emetic toxin

1. Introduction

Bacillus cereus (sensu lato) is a member of the Bacillus genus which currently includes *Bacillus mycoides, Bacillus pseudomycoides, Bacillus weihenstephanensis, Bacillus anthracis, Bacillus thuringiensis, B. cereus sensu stricto* (usually called *B. cereus*), *B. cytotoxicus* and *B. toyonensis.* Newly identified species have been isolated from marine sediments and other environments and added to this group: *B. paranthracis, B. pacificus, B. tropicus, B. albus, B. mobilis, B. luti, B. proteolyticus, B. nitratireducens* and *B. paramycoides*, with some other strains that under evaluation [1]. *B. cereus* is very closely related to *B. anthracis* and *B. thuringiensis*, and it has been proposed that *B. anthracis* is a lineage of *B. cereus* [2]. There is significant research interest in *B. cereus* and *B. anthracis* due to the pathogenicity of both species and there have been reported cases of *B. cereus* causing anthrax-like diseases [3, 4].

Bacillus cereus is a toxin-producing, endospore-forming, gram-positive, and facultative bacterium which is ubiquitous in the environment, and often found associated

IntechOpen

with soil, growing plants, and in the intestinal tract of animals [5–8]. Its ability to form spores allows this organism to persist in the environment regardless of environmental conditions that are not favorable to growth [9]. Regarding food products, this bacterium has been isolated from air in a cow shed [10], rice, spices, milk and dairy products, vegetables, meat, farinaceous foods, desserts, and cakes [9].

This organism is a major problem to the food industry because it is difficult to eliminate from food products due to its ability to survive in different environments despite environmental stresses which would normally inhibit bacterial survival [11], spore resistance to heat, dehydration, acid, and other physical stresses, and an inability to be destroyed through pasteurization and other sanitation procedures [5, 12]. It is estimated that (1.4–12%) of all food poisoning in the world is related to *B. cereus* [13]. There are two types of food poisoning, emetic syndrome and diarrheal syndrome, which have been described. However, this organism is known to cause a variety of other clinical infections such as local infections, such as in burns, traumatic wounds, and the eye, bacteremia and septicemia, central nervous system infection (meningitis, abscesses, and shunt-associated infections), respiratory infections, endocarditis and pericarditis, endophthalmitis, periodontitis, and osteomyelitis [12, 14, 15].

Emetic syndrome is caused by a cereulide which is a heat-stable peptide toxin. Diarrheal syndrome is caused by a host of other enterotoxins produced by the organism including nonhemolytic enterotoxin (NHE), enterotoxin FM (EntFM), Hemolysin BL (HBL), and cytotoxin K (Cyt K) [14, 16]. Hemolysin BL has consisted of three different components; one bending component B (encoded by hblA gene) and two lytic components L1 and L2 (encoded by hblC and hblD genes) [12]. Nausea and are symptoms of emetic syndrome, which usually occurs 1–5 hours after ingestion of contaminated food [16]. Diarrheal syndrome results in abdominal pain and diarrheal 8 to 16 hours post-ingestion [5, 14]. These illnesses are generally short-lived and self-resolve within 24 hours [17].

Bacillus cereus is underreported as a food-borne pathogen. First, symptoms of disease are usually mild and transitory. Second, since it is ubiquitous in the environment, there is not a direct linkage of animals to human infection, such as *Escherichia coli* or *Salmonella*, thus it is often ignored. Third, emetic strains are not detected using standard methods for *B. cereus* such as the use of mannitol-egg yolk-polymyxin agar (MYP). Finally, the food sources that are involved in food poisoning outbreaks contain different *B. cereus* strains [18]. Nevertheless, there have been multiple outbreaks caused by *B. cereus*. Between 1998 and 2000 *B. cereus* was the cause of 60% of foodborne outbreaks in mass catering facilities, and it was the most frequently isolated microorganism from commercial kitchen samples [5]. In 2014, 287 outbreaks of food poisoning were due to *B. cereus* resulting in 3073 cases, and in 2015, 291 outbreaks resulting in 3131 cases were reported in European Member States [17]. An investigation found that *B. cereus* was responsible for 1689 food poisoning cases at mass-catering services in the European Union from 2000 to 2013 [17]. Another study provided strong evidence that *B. cereus* caused 564 foodborne illness outbreaks in France from 2007 to 2014 [19]. Bennett et al. reported that 235 food-borne outbreaks, involving 2050 illnesses and 17 cases hospitalizations were caused by *Bacillus cereus* in the United States between 1998 and 2008 [20].

Given the prevalence of *B. cereus* in food products, its pathogenicity, and the impact of *B. cereus* on the worldwide foodborne illness burden, it is imperative to improve control and detection of this pathogen in food. We aim to summarize what is currently known about *B. cereus*, discuss current research into control and detection of this pathogen, and identify research that needs to be conducted to reduce the presence of this pathogen in food.

2. Biological properties of *Bacillus cereus*

Bacillus cereus is a mesophilic bacterium and is widespread in the environment. It grows at temperatures ranging from 4 to 48°C, with optimal growth temperatures of 28–35°C. One study divided *B. cereus* isolates into two groups dependent on their growth temperature range; a low-temperature range of 4 to 37°C and a high-temperature range 10 to 42°C [21]. It is salt tolerant to 7.5% w/w concentrations and to a pH range of 4.5 to 9.5 [21–23]. The minimum water activity for growth is 0.93 [21, 24].

Bacillus cereus cells are rod shape and measure approximately 1.0–1.2 μm in width by 3.0–5.0 μm in length. Its colonies measure 3–8 mm which appear as grayish flat colonies with a ground glass-like appearance, and often rough edges. *Bacillus cereus* spores have an ellipsoidal or cylindrical shape, look green in a red vegetative cytoplasm cell, and include black lipid globules in intracellular lipid stain. Spores do not cause swelling in the sporangium [24, 25]. Chemical analysis of *Bacillus cereus* shows that it can make acid from glucose but not from mannitol, xylose, and arabinose [22]. Its oxidase test is negative, while its motility, catalase, citrate utilization, casein hydrolysis, nitrate reduction, and Voges-Proskauer (VP) reaction, l-tyrosine reduction, and growth in 0.001% lysozyme tests are positive [24, 25].

3. Pathogenicity of *Bacillus cereus*

Pathogenicity of *B. cereus* is based on its potential to colonize and persist in the host and invade tissues [26]. This ability varies from strain to strain, which makes it hard to understand and administrate the risks associated with *B. cereus* [1]. Although *B. cereus* is known to cause other diseases, such as respiratory tract infections, nosocomial infections, endophthalmtis, and central nervous system infections, we will be focusing on its role in foodborne illness [7].

Ultimately, food poisoning from *B. cereus* is due to its presence in food. Its presence may initially causes changes in the texture of food and the development of off-flavors due to the production of toxins and/or reproduction of vegetative cells [22]. After consumption of contaminated food, two main types of food poisoning may occur; emetic syndrome or diarrheal syndrome. High microbial count are required before toxin production begins, thus the infective dose of *B. cereus* is 10^5 to 10^7 for diarrheal disease and 10^5 to 10^8 cell/g for the emetic syndrome [27, 28]. Therefore, a consensus exists regarding the dose of *B. cereus* which is necessary to make the food safe for consumption and should not surpass the 10^3 CFU/g [22].

3.1 Diarrheal syndrome

Diarrheal food poisoning was recognized in 1948 for the first time after a food poisoning outbreak in Oslo, Norway [29]. In 1955, Hauge voluntarily conducted an experiment and ingested vanilla sauce with a high number of *B. cereus* which subsequently resulted in abdominal pain and diarrhea. This experiment indicated that *B. cereus* infection can result in diarrheal disease. Toxins are produced by the bacteria in the small intestine when growth has reached the phase between exponential and stationary phases [25]. Three different heat-labile toxins are responsible for this syndrome: hemolysin BL (HBL), non-hemolytic enterotoxin (Nhe), and cytotoxin K (CytK). As mentioned before, HBL constitutes three protein complexes, L_1, L_2, and B (encoded by genes hblD, hblC, and hblA, respectively). This enterotoxin is cytotoxic and has hemolytic ability, which is the ability to destroy red blood cells by forming transmembrane pores. Additionally, activation of adenylate cyclase enzymes is another mechanism used to cause diarrheal disease [25, 30].

Nhe is another cytotoxic enterotoxin that has three protein components, NheA, NheB, and NheC, which are encoded by the genes nheA, nheB, and nheC. NheB is a cell binding protein,, while nheC acts as a catalyst for bringing nheA and nheB together. This enterotoxin was discovered after a Norwegian outbreak that was caused by a strain that did not produce the HBL enterotoxin. It resembles HBL structurally, and both HBL and Nhe are similar in that they need all three components to be biologically active [25, 27, 30].

In contrast, Cytotoxin K (CytK) is a single protein encoded by gene cytK which is another b-barrel pore-forming toxin. About 90% of *B. cereus* strains may have the gene for this toxin. Similar to other b-barrel pore-forming toxins, it creates oligomers that are susceptible to boiling and resistant to sodium dodecyl sulfate (SDS). It has two forms, CytK-1 and CytK-2 which have an 89% amino acid sequence similarity. The first form is more involved in French necrotic enteritis outbreaks [25, 30], for which fatal cases have been reported from ref. [31]. Each of these single enterotoxins could cause diarrheal symptoms individually [25].

The enterotoxins are produced in a temperature range of (10–43°C) with an optimum of 32°C. Toxins are susceptible to heat, rapidly degraded at pH 3, and hydrolyzed by proteolytic enzymes of the digestive tract. This shows that diarrheal syndrome is caused by ingestion of cells or spores rather than of produced toxins, however, in young people, both preformed toxin and ingestion of cells can cause diarrheal food poisoning because those people do not have enough stomach acid to destroy the toxins [25]. This syndrome results in a mild and watery diarrhea disease that is similar to the diarrheal syndrome caused by *Clostridium perfringens.* Most individuals suffering from diarrheal disease recover within 24 h without any treatment [1, 30].

3.2 Emetic syndrome

Emetic syndrome is also caused by *B. cereus*, is more acute than diarrheal syndrome, and has a shorter incubation time. Consumption of toxin results in vomiting, nausea, and abdominal cramps 1 to 6 h after ingestion of contaminated food. When cell populations reach 10^5–10^8 cells per gram sufficient toxin is produced in the food for causing this syndrome [30]. The main cause of this syndrome is cereulide toxin [1]. Some experiments relying on monkey feeding showed that the causative dose of cereulide toxin is 70 μg for this syndrome [25]. Cereulide is not eliminated by cooking or digestive processes since it is both heat and acid stable [18].

This is a nonribosomal peptide that is encoded by the 24-kb cereulide synthetase of genes (ces). Cereulide acts as a potassium ionophore and decomposes the transmembrane potential which results in mitochondrial inactivation and human natural killer cell inhibition by stimulating swelling and respiration. It can also causes degeneration of hepatocytes in higher dose [27]. This syndrome occurs when the pre-formed toxin binds to 5-HT_3 receptors and stimulates the vomiting center of the brain in a way similar to Staphylococcus enterotoxins. Because of its similarity to *Staphylococcus* enterotoxins, it is very hard to distinguish the symptoms [25].

Cereulide is produced in the stationary growth phase of *B. cereus* in food at a temperature range of 12–37°C and wth an ideal temperature of 12–15°C. [25]. Cereulide production is produced in foods with $a_w > 0.953$ and pH of >5.6, under aerobic conditions, when more than 10^6 CFU of *B. cereus* emetic strains are present in each gram of food [27].

The prevalence of emetic strains of *B. cereus* is high in nonrandom food and clinical samples (32.8%), compared to the overall prevalence in *B. cereus* isolates. Still, 4.7% of ice cream, 1.6% of fish products, 11.0% of ready-to-eat foods, 3.9% of other food samples not implicated in food poisoning, 1.7% of soil samples, 1.5% of cow milk, 1.2% of cow bedding, and 3.9% of farm rinsing water samples contained *B. cereus* emetic strain isolates [18].

4. Toxins of *Bacillus cereus*

B. cereus produces different virulence factors including phospholipases, hemolysins, and enterotoxins [32]. One emetic toxin and three enterotoxins are the causative agent for the associated food poisonings [33]. The Emetic toxin is produced in food stuff and three enterotoxins that are responsible for diarrheal syndrome are produced in intestine [34].

4.1 Emetic toxin (cereulide)

In 1976, Melling et al. proposed for the first time that a different toxin is associated with emetic syndrome. They proposed this by feeding Rhesus monkey with two different isolated strains: one from a diarrheal associated outbreak and another one from a vomiting associated outbreaks. The first strain caused fluid accumulation while the second one did not. This indicated that a different toxin is involved in vomiting symptoms [35]. Then, Agata et al. [36], identified cereulide as the emetic toxin factor [36].

Cereulide is a ring-structured peptide (dodecadepsipeptide) which is constituted of three repeat sequences of four amino acids and/or oxy-acids. Its molecular weight is 1.2 kDa and its composition is [d-O-leu-d-ala-l-O-val-l-val] [25, 27]. This potassium binding depsipeptide is structurally similar to the ionophore valinomycin. Its lipophilic properties, as well as heat and pH resistance, are due to its structure which is characterized by peptide and ester bonds. It is not eliminated by bactofugation or filtration, nor by heat treatments (even at 121°C for 2 hours) in food processing. Also, pepsin and trypsin in the stomach do not have a lethal effect on it. Therefore, it is very important to control cereulide production. Some food additives such as polyphosphates could be effective for this purpose, while other food ingredients motivate its production [33]. It has seven different isoforms named isocereulide A-G [37], which have different cytotoxicity. Isocereulide-A, the highly cytotoxic isocereulide [37], has 10-fold cytotoxicity compared to wild cereulide type, while isocereulide-B has no cytotoxicity. This difference is due to the different membrane activity of the isocereulide [33].

Foodborne disease caused by cereulide results in heavy episodes of vomiting, while recently more severe intoxications show rhabdomyolysis, liver damage, and serious multi-organ failures. This is because of its high ionophoric activity [33]. A 17 year old boy died after consuming spaghetti with pesto that was prepared 4 days earlier. Within 2 days of having the meal, the boy developed fulminant liver failure and rhabdomyolysis which resulted in his death [38].

It is also reported that cereulide can co-occur with other microbial toxins in cereal-based foods such as mycotoxins [33]. A research by Agata et al. [39], quantified the production of *B. cereus* emetic toxin (cereulide) in various foods. In 13 out of 14 food samples that were involved in emetic type food-poisoning, cereulide was identified at a range of 0.01 to 1.28 μg per 1 g food. An emetic producing strain of *B. cereus* (*B. cereus* NC7401), was identified as the causative agent [39].

Considering *B. cereus* is ubiquitous in the environment, the emetic toxin is not produced in large amount in foods. A research study evaluated 271 samples of soil, animal feces, raw and processed vegetables, concluded that while *B. cereus* is common in the environment, the incidence of emetic strains of *B. cereus* is rare [40].

Carlin et al. [41] evaluated 100 strains of *B. cereus* to see if emetic toxin producing strains have different characteristics than non-emetic toxin-producing strains. Among them, 17 strains were emetic toxin (cereulide) producing and 83 strains non-emetic toxin-producing. The minimum growth temperature of emetic toxin-producing strains is 10°C and maximum of 48°C, while 11% of non-emetic toxin-producing strains grow at 4°C and 47% of them at 7°C and only 39% of them can grow at 48°C. Spores from emetic toxin-producing strains have higher resistance at temperatures of 90°C and lower germination rate at 7°C than other strains. This study indicates that emetic toxin-producing strains have different growth characteristics than other strains, which is useful for *B. cereus* risk assessment [41]. Another investigation showed that all cereulide producing strains contain the H-1 serovar phenotype, while non-emetic toxin producing group does not show this phenotype. The H-1 serovar group is enable to hydrolyze starch, thus the emetic toxin-producing strains cannot hydrolyze starch. This may help to control outbreaks of emetic type syndrome caused by *B. cereus* [42].

4.2 Enterotoxins

In the late 1970s and early 1980s researcher started to isolate enterotoxins. An unstable, and heat-labile protein, which was inactivated in 30 min at 56°C, was isolated for the first time as an enterotoxin protein. Then it was reported that diarrheal activity of *B. cereus* is caused by a complex of two or three protein enterotoxin [12]. Three different enterotoxins have been identified that are produced by *B. cereus*. Studies show *B. cereus* produces one single-component enterotoxin and two different three-component enterotoxins [6].

4.2.1 Hemolytic BL (Hbl)

Hbl is an eneterotoxin that was originally highly purified *from B. cereus* F837/ 76. [12]. It is a three-component enterotoxin containing two-lytic components, L_2, L_1, and binding (B) compound, which is encoded by the Hbl operon by hblC, hblD, and hblA respectively. Two different Hbl operons exist in some *B. cereus* strains, with the most common one containing a fourth gene, hblB. This gene encodes the Hbl bind compound precursor HblB'. The molecular weights of the components are 45, 36, and 35 kDa for L_2, L_1, and B, respectively [33], and 5.3 pI value [12]. Hbl has been identified in 42–73% of food poisoning strains and less frequent in non-pathogenic strains [43].

Evaluation of all three components of Hbl revealed that the proteins formed alpha-helices. Analysis of Hbl-B and L_1 contained transmembrane segments of 17 amino acids and 60 amino acids residues respectively, whereas L_2 did not contain any transmembrane domains. [12]. For biological activity of hbl, all three components are needed [43]. Hb has hemolytic activity as evidenced byring-shaped clearing zones due to hemolysis on blood agar. The hemolytic potential is based on the type of blood used in the experiment. Besides hemolytic activity, hbl increases vascular permeability in rabbit skin and is dermonecrotic. Cytotoxicity has also exhibited toxicity to Chinese hamster ovary cells and retinal tissue. In addition to fluid accumulation in the rabbit ileal loop assay, it causes pore formation in eukaryotic cell membranes [12]. Of note, hbl needs to be combined with nhe to be active biologically [43].

Heterogeneity exists in the hbl components in different strains. Schoeni and Wong [44], studied 127 *B. cereus* isolates and results showed that across all isolates there were only four variations of the B subunit(38, 42, 44, and 46 kDa), two different L_1 subunits (38 and 41 kDa), and three different L_2 subunits (43, 45, and 49 kDa) [44].

4.2.2 Non-hemolytic enterotoxin (Nhe)

Granum et al. [29], found that there should be one enterotoxin in addition to hemolysin BL and enterotoxin T that is responsible for diarrheal syndrome, after evaluating 321 strains of *B. cereus* [29]. While evaluating *B. cereus* strain 0075-95, isolated from a Norwegian outbreak, Nhe was purified for the first time [45]. This is also a three component open reading frame that is encoded by *nheA, nheB,* and *nheC.* Their molecular weights are 41, 39.8, and 36.5 kDa with a pI value of 5.13, 5.61, and 5.28 for *nheA, nheB,* and *nheC* respectively [12]. Also, *nheA, nheB,* and *nheC* have signal peptides of 26, 30, and 30 amino acids, mature proteins of 360, 372, and 329 amino acids, respectively [46].

Nhe protein components have similarities with each other as well as with hbl protein components. *NheA* has 19% similarity with *nheB,* and *nheC*, also *nheB* has 44% similarity with *nheC*. The similarities between nhe and hbl components are observed as 24% between *nheA* and L_2, 37% between *nheB* and L_1, and 25% between *nheC* and B [12, 46]. Some homologies also exist between nhe and hbl regarding the predicted transmembrane helices, in that hbl and nhe are a tripartite family [8, 12].

About 92 to 100% of *B. cereus* isolates produce nhe toxin, which is found more often than hbl production [12]. This shows that nhe is the most dominant toxin in diarrheal food poisoning, demonstrating that cytotoxicity of *B. cereus* is greatly related to the concentration of nhe and poorly to the concentration of hbl [47]. Studies revealed that no change in cytotoxicity was observed after inhibition of hbl and cytK in *B. thuringiensis*, while deletion of nhe operon in *B. cereus* strain ATCC 14579 reduced cytotoxicity activity [8].

The biological activities of nhe are based on the involvement of all three components of nhe. Nhe exhibits a a specific concentration of ratio of (10:10:1 for nheA:nheB:nheC) [33]. Though the mode of action of nhe is not completely clear, the disruption of the plasma membrane and pore formation in planar lipid bilayers were observed in epithelia [47]. This result shows that nhe causes cell death (cytotoxicity) via colloid osmotic lysis by forming transmembrane pores. Also, suspension assays indicate hemolytic activity of nhe toward erythrocytes [8].

4.2.3 Cytotoxin K (cytK)

This is a single protein diarrheal enterotoxin that was isolated in 1998 from *B. cereus* strain NVH 391/98. This strain caused a severe bloody diarrheal outbreak in France that resulted in six cases and three deaths. CytK toxin is encoded by *cytK*, which has two variants, *cytK-1*, and *cytK-2*, with 89% amino acid similarity [33]. In 2015, Castiaux et al. conducted a research study to determine whether cytK is a virulence factor for diarrheal syndrome. Results showed that cytK-2 is not a relevant virulence factor for this type of food poisoning [48]. Another study also declared that cytK-2 is not a good marker for the cytotoxicity of *B. cereus* [33].

This toxin is a member of the β-folded pore-forming group and has different health effects [49]. CytK-1 is a hemolytic, dermonecrotic, pore-forming in lipid layers, and highly toxic to the human intestinal epithelial cells. CytK-2 also proved to be hemolytic, cytotoxic, and pore-forming in lipid layers, but has about 80% lower cytotoxicity power than cytK-1 [33, 49]. Shadrin et al. [49], observed the cytK genes of some *B. cereus* strains and concluded that there is a distinct differentiation between cytK-1 and cytK-2. Thus, by knowing the variants of cytk in a strain, we can recognize if cytk is the main cause of extreme diarrheal disease [49]. A duplex PCR assay was developed to discriminate *B. cereus* strains carrying the cytK-1 gene. This was the first recognized method for identifying the strains containing this gene [50].

4.2.4 Enterotoxin FM (entFM)

This toxin is the most prevalent enterotoxin in *B. cereus,* and was identified from the *B. cereus* FM1 strain by Asano in 1997. PCR studies of 10 *B. cereus* isolates showed the presence of the entFM gene in all isolated strains [51, 52]. Another study revealed the presence of the entFM gene in 27 of 28 food isolates and 30 outbreaks associated with *B. cereus* strains [53]. In another study, the entFM gene was detected in all 616 strains of *B. cereus* and *B. thuringiensis* [54]. Therefore, because of its prevalence in approximately all *B. cereus* strains, it can be a target gene for assessing enterotoxigenic *B. cereus* isolates [51].

Although the majority of investigated strains were positive for entFM, only a small number of them could cause diarrheal toxicity. This may be due to the expression level of the entFM gene [51]. Research studies showed that entFM is related to cell wall peptidase (Cwps) which is involved in bacterial motility, shape, and biofilm formation, as well as vacuolization of macrophages as part of bacterial virulence [52].

There have been other identified enterotoxins produced by *B. cereus*, but little is known about their virulence and mode of action (**Table 1**).

Toxin Name	Toxin Type	Molecular Weight	pI	References
Cereulide	Emetic toxin	1.2 kDa	5.52	[55, 56]
Hemolytic BL	Enterotoxin	37–46 kDa	5.3	[12, 55]
B-component		35 kDa	5.34	[33, 57]
L1-component		36 kDa	5.33	[33, 57]
L2-component		45 kDa	5.33	[33, 57]
Non-hemolytic	Enterotoxin	36–41 kDa	5.13	[55]
nheA		41 kDa	5.61	[12]
nheB		39.8 kDa	5.28	[12]
nheC		36.5 kDa		[12]
Cytotoxin K	Enterotoxin	34 kDa	6.1	[31, 55]

Table 1.
Molecular size and isoelectric point of toxins produced by B. cereus.

Antibiotics	*B. cereus* **reaction to antibiotics**		
	Susceptible	**Intermediate**	**Resistant**
Amoxicillin/Clavulanic Acid	–	–	+
Ampicillin	–	–	+
Benzyl Penicillin	–	–	+
Cefepime	–	–	+
Cefotaxime*	–	–	+
Cefoxitin	–	–	+
Cefpodoxime	–	–	+
Ceftazidime	–	–	+
Cloxacillin	–	–	+
Cotrimoxazole**	–	–	+
Cephalothin	–	–	+
Metronidazole	–	–	+
Nalidixic Acid	–	–	+
Nitrofurantoin	–	–	+
Novobiocin	–	–	+
Oxacillin	–	–	+
Penicillin G	–	–	+
Rifampicin***	–	–	+
Trimethoprim	–	–	+
Amikacin	+	–	–
Azithromycin	+	–	–
Chloramphenicol	+	–	–
Ciprofloxacin	+	–	–
Clindamycin	+	–	–
Erythromycin	+	–	–
Gentamicin	+	–	–
Imipenem	+	–	–
Kanamycin	+	–	–
Moxifloxacin	+	–	–
Telithromycin	+	–	–
Tetracycline	+	–	–
Sulfamethoxazole	+	–	–
Vancomycin	+		–
Ceftriaxone	–	+	–
Streptomycin	–	+	–

*Natural resistance to beta-lactams.
**66% resistant.
***Acquired resistance phenotype.

Table 2.
B. cereus antibiotic resistance [61, 66–69].

5. Antibiotic resistance of *Bacillus cereus*

Antibiotic resistance is a process by which microorganisms show tolerance against antibiotics that are used to treat people from diseases [58]. The growing number of antibiotic-resistant microorganisms have been reported as a major health problem in the twenty-first century. Therefore, several investigations have investigated this topic and revealed information about the antibiotic resistance potential of microorganisms [59]. Antibiotic resistance of *B. cereus* has been tested in different food products and reported in different studies.

Fiedler et all. In 2019, evaluated the antibiotic resistance of 147 *B. cereus* strains isolated from fresh vegetables including cucumbers, carrots, herbs, salad leaves, and ready-to-eat mixed salad leaves. It shows that *B. cereus* is highly resistant to β-lactam antibiotics such as penicillin G (PEN) and cefotaxime (CTX) (100%), ampicillin (AMP), and amoxicillin/clavulanic acid combination (AMC) (99.3%). This study showed these isolates were still is susceptible to ciprofloxacin (CIP) (99.3%), chloramphenicol (CHL) (98.6%), amikacin (AMK) (98.0%), imipenem (IPM) (93.9%), erythromycin (ERY) (91.8%), gentamicin (GEN) (88.4%), tetracycline (TET) (76.2%), and trimethoprim-sulfamethoxazole (SXT) (52.4%) [59]. Another study assessed the antibiotic resistance of 64 *B. cereus* strains isolated from different food products such as milk, dairy products, spices, and rice salad in Morocco. This investigation indicated that isolated strains are resistant to ampicillin (98.4%), tetracycline (90.6%), oxacillin (100%), cefepime (100%), and penicillin (100%), and were susceptible to chloramphenicol (67.2%), erythromycin (84.4%), and gentamicin (100%) [60]. These data are in concordance with other investigations in [61–65]. Most of these studies were performed using the Kirby-Bauer disc diffusion method for testing antibiotic resistance of the *B. cereus* isolates (**Table 2**).

6. Detection methods of *Bacillus cereus*

Because of *B. cereus'* high incidence, and its wide distribution in food and the environment, its detection is very important for recognizing pathogenic *B. cereus* strains and preventing food contamination and food-poisoning outbreaks [70]. Different factors are considered in developing detection techniques for *B. cereus* including, sensitivity, usage, and time. Therefore, to have useful techniques to detect *B. cereus* cells and spores from a low level of contamination, several detection methods have been developed.

6.1 Traditional methods

Agar plate-based counting (ISO 7932:2004) is a traditional method for detection and detection of *B. cereus* [1]. For detection and enumeration of low numbers of bacteria using the most probable number, ISO 21,871 has been used. The result of traditional methods was presented as "presumptive *B. cereus*" because these methods could not evaluate the toxin-producing ability of *B. cereus* and could not differentiate *B. cereus* from other Bacillus group isolates [71]. Therefore, after doing several laboratories steps, a differentiative method needed to be performed to complete the detection process and differentiate *B. cereus* from other Bacillus group bacteria [1]. These detection techniques were based on the use of selective media and biochemical tests, which are arduous, time-consuming, and need skilled personnel to perform [70]. Thus, novel techniques have to be developed to narrow these gaps.

6.2 Molecular methods

Since low levels of contamination might be present in food, a very sensitive method needs to be used to detect low numbers of *B. cereus* rapidly. The polymerase chain reaction (PCR) is a fast and sensitive method that can be used to determine the enterotoxic potential of *B. cereus* [72]. The PCR method was developed to identify different pathogenic bacteria. Nested PCR, Randomly Amplified Polymorphic DNA PCR (RAPD PCR), quantitative PCR (qPCR), and multiplex PCR (mPCR) [70] are different molecular techniques that have been developed. Traditional PCR uses a pair of primers to produce a nucleic acid fragment and can only be applied for a single pathogenic factor. Multiplex PCR uses more two or more pairs of primers to detect multiple pathogenic factors [73].

A research study was performed to compare multiplex PCR, enzyme immunoassay, and cell culture methods for detection of enterotoxigenic *B. cereus*. They assessed 176 strains of *B. cereus* from different sources and the results obtained from these three methods were correlated. The PCR assay was suggested as a convenient method for the detection of enterotoxigenic *B. cereus* isolates [74]. Another study investigated a novel method of antibiotic-based magnetic nanoprobes combined with mPCR for the detection of *B. cereus* as well as *Staphylococcus aureus*. In this study, more than one pathogen can be detected, unlike other methods that are designed for the detection of one pathogen (for detail refer to [73]). This study indicates the advantages of the PCR method when used with other methods in the detection process.

These methods are mainly based on specific gene sequences, which can result in false negatives due to improper cell disruption and nucleic acid extraction. Thus, on a small scale it is not necessarily an easy, real-time and rapid detection method for *B. cereus* [70], however, it has advantages compared to the traditional plating methods such as shorter time overall and higher specificity [1]. These methods are unlikely to be used by the food industry as it requires professionals well-trained in molecular techniques [1] Additionally, molecular methods experience detection interference from complex foodstuff which decreases their sensitivity [73]. Therefore, to overcome these limitations new biosensors techniques have been developed.

6.3 Biosensors methods

Over the last year, biosensors are the most reliable developed methods for the detection of pathogens [1]. This is due to their simplicity, rapidity, and high sensitivity [71]. Additionally, this technique needs a small number of samples to work [1]. Different biosensor techniques have been developed for which DNA-based [1] and electrochemical-based [71] are reported as the best biosensor methods.

Poly and monoclonal antibodies are used as diagnostic factors in biosensors as an alternative to DNA probes [1]. Enzyme-linked immunosorbent assay (ELISA) is a sensitive and convenient method for assessing the macromolecular protein, polysaccharide, and bacteria. This method is based on two antibodies, monoclonal antibody (mAb) and rabbit polyclonal antibody, and it is a rapid detection method for low numbers of cells ($9 * 10^2$ cells/mL). Immunological kits are commercially available, like the *B. cereus* Enterotoxin Test Kit, but they cannot be used on whole-cells. For detection of whole cells, sandwich ELISA is best for identification of *B. cereus* even in low concentrations [70].

The antibody-based assays have some disadvantages, such as being costly, because commercial *B. cereus* antibodies are expensive, have low affinity, and pH and temperature can affect their stability and binding potential [1]. To inhibit these disadvantages, bacteriophage and their proteins can be used as recognition elements instead of antibodies because they have high sensitivity, high binding affinity, and high stability to temperature and pH [75].

7. Control of *Bacillus cereus*

B. cereus endospores are very heat-resistant spores that survive cooking proccesses. Heat resistance increases with an increase of salinity and decreases as acidity increases [76]. Some improper food preparation methods, increase the risk of pathogens' growth such as improper cooling methods [77]. A survey of 411 schools indicated that 78% of schools cool leftover food which is later heated and served at another meal. Only 8% of schools use blast chillers, and many cool food using improper cooling methods [78], which can allow for *B. cereus* to proliferate. Therefore, standard operating procedures are necessary to prevent *B. cereus* associated food-poisoning outbreaks.

Schneider et al. [76], reported best practices for controlling *B. cereus* outgrowth in food products. These recommendations were based on the National Institutes of Health (NIH), the National Institute of Allergy and Infectious Diseases (NIAID), the National Food Processors Association (NFPA), and the FDA Food Code 2013, that are effective for destroying *B. cereus*:

- Steaming the food in ≥145°F (63°C) under pressure, roasting, frying, and grilling methods can destroy *B. cereus* vegetative cells and spores.

- To inhibit the emetic toxin, foods need to be heated to 249°F (121°C) for more than 80 minutes.

- Cooking to ≥145°F (63°C) and reheating to 165°F (74°C) for 15 seconds destroy the vegetative cells. While, if the toxin has been preformed in food, it is not safe to eat.

- The quick cooling of foods after heating is the best way to prevent spores from erminating.

- For spore formation inhibition, hot foods should be kept at 135°F (57°C) and cold foods below 41°F (5°C).

- Cool or refrigerate leftovers rapidly to 41°F (5°C) or below.

Additional methods have been investigated for control of *B. cereus* in food. A study by Luu-Thi et al. [79] looked at the use of high pressure high temperature (HPHT) treatments for control of *B. cereus*. Spore inactivation was less than 1-log at 50–60°C but increased to 5-log at 100°C [79]. Their studies using the antimicoribial carvacrol in conjunction of HPHT showed reduced inactivation of spores at temperatures under 90°C and did not have an affect at 95–100°C.

Studies using combinations of radiation and antimicrobials were performed by Ayari et al. [80]. The use of carvacrol in combination of nisin enhanced radiation sensitivity and resulted in lower D_{10} values [80]. However, repeated exposure to

1 kGy of γ-radiation resulted in an increase in radioresistance indicating that repeated exposures would be ineffective for control in food products.

Studies conducted by Yang et al. [81] looked at the use of lactic acid bacteria (LAB) starter cultures in rice fermentations as a way to control *B. cereus* [81]. With the decrease in pH from 6.8 to 4.0 there was a 1 log cfu/ml reduction in *B. cereus*. These results are consistent with results obtained by Rossland et al. [82] which showed varying results in feremented milk ranging from a 7-log reduction to as little as a 2-log reduction [82]. These results indicate that use of LAB may produce inconsistent results and may not inhibit *B. cereus* sufficiently to insure safety of food products.

Studies were conducted to look at the use of bactericidal activity of neutral electrolyzed water (NEW) against *B. cereus* inoculated onto the surface of fresh produce items (cherry tomato, miniature cucumber, carrot and parsley) and polypropylene cutting boards at ambient temperature (22°C). NEW solutions contained 60 and 120 mg/L free available chlorine (FAC). When used on cell suspensions 5 min of treatment a 2.11 to 3.03 $\log_{10}$ CFU/mL reduction of *B. cereus* was observed [83]. *B. cereus* on inoculated produce was reduced by 2.11–2.30 and 2.41–3.16 $\log_{10}$ CFU/g when NEW contained 120 mg/L FAC. On surfaces, after 5 mins of treatment, cell viability was reduced by 2.33 and 3.06 $\log_{10}$ per 100 cm^2. These results indicated that a pre-treatment with NEW containing FAC may be a method to further investigate for pre-treatment of food products to protect against outgrowth of *B. cereus*.

8. Conclusion

B. cereus is an endospore-forming bacterium that is ubiquitous in the environment and can be isolated from different foods. Its spores are strongly resistant to heat, acid, and other environmental stresses. This makes contamination of *B. cereus* a concern as a food pathogen. Since illness with *B. cereus* are often a short duration and self-limiting, illnesses from *B. cereus* are underestimated.

Emetic and diarrheal syndromes are the two types of food-borne diseases caused by *B. cereus*. Cereulide toxin which is formed in food is the cause of the emetic syndrome and different enterotoxins including HBL, NHE, cytK, and entFM are the cause of the diarrheal syndrome. This bacterium is resistant to some antibiotics such as the β-lactam group and susceptible to some other antibiotics like gentamicin (GEN). It is unknown if antimicrobial resistance is increasing in *B. cereus*, but this needs further investigation given the number of antibiotics that *B. cereus* is resistant to.

Different detection methods are used for identifying pathogenic *B. cereus* strains to help prevent food contamination. However, there are limitations to current rapid detection of *B. cereus* especially given its fgenetic similarity to *Bacillus anthracis*, *Bacillus thuringiensis*, and *Bacillus mycoides* [84, 85]. Moreover, molecular detection methods require costly instrumentation and are not likely to be accessible by the majority of food processors. Therefore, different molecular techniques are needed to differentiate these bacteria from each other, and rapid tests that can be utilized by industry are needed.

Current control practices, as defined by FDA and other regulatory agencies are not adequate for eliminating *B. cereus* from food. Research into new methods to control or eliminate *B. cereus* from food products is desperately needed.

Conflict of interest

The authors declare no conflict of interest.

Author details

Barakatullah Mohammadi, Natasha Gorkina and Stephanie A. Smith*
Washington State University, Pullman, WA, USA

*Address all correspondence to: steph.smith@wsu.edu

IntechOpen

© 2022 The Author(s). Licensee IntechOpen. This chapter is distributed under the terms of the Creative Commons Attribution License (http://creativecommons.org/licenses/by/3.0), which permits unrestricted use, distribution, and reproduction in any medium, provided the original work is properly cited.

References

[1] Ramarao N, Tran SL, Marin M, Vidic J. Advanced methods for detection of *Bacillus cereus* and its pathogenic factors. Sensors. 2020;**20**(9):1-23. DOI: 10.3390/s20092667

[2] Helgason E et al. *Bacillus anthracis*, *Bacillus cereus*, and *Bacillus thuringiensis*—One species on the basis of genetic evidence. Applied and Environmental Microbiology. 2000;**66**(6):2627-2630. DOI: 10.1128/AEM.66.6.2627-2630.2000

[3] Liu Y et al. Proposal of nine novel species of the *Bacillus cereus* group. International Journal of Systematic and Evolutionary Microbiology. 2017;**67**(8):2499-2508. DOI: 10.1099/ijsem.0.001821

[4] Baldwin VM. You Can't *B. cereus*—A review of *Bacillus cereus* strains that cause Anthrax-like disease. Frontiers in Microbiology. 2020;**11**(August):1-16. DOI: 10.3389/fmicb.2020.01731

[5] Ehling-Schulz M, Knutsson R, Scherer S. *Bacillus cereus*. Genomes of Foodborne and Waterborne Pathogens. 2010:147-164. DOI: 10.1128/9781555816902.ch11

[6] Granum PE, Lund T. *Bacillus cereus* and its food poisoning toxins. FEMS Microbiology Letters. 1997;**157**(2):223-228. DOI: 10.1016/S0378-1097(97)00438-2

[7] Bottone EJ. *Bacillus cereus*, a volatile human pathogen. Clinical Microbiology Reviews. 2010;**23**(2):382-398. DOI: 10.1128/CMR.00073-09

[8] Stenfors Arnesen LP, Fagerlund A, Granum PE. From soil to gut: *Bacillus cereus* and its food poisoning toxins. FEMS Microbiology Reviews. 2008;**32**(4):579-606. DOI: 10.1111/j.1574-6976.2008.00112.x

[9] Ghelardi E, Celandroni F, Salvetti S, Barsotti C, Baggiani A, Senesi S. Identification and characterization of toxigenic *Bacillus cereus* isolates responsible for two food-poisoning outbreaks. FEMS Microbiology Letters. 2002;**208**(1):129-134. DOI: 10.1016/S0378-1097(02)00450-0

[10] Ehling-Schulz M, Lereclus D, Koehler TM. The *Bacillus cereus* group: Bacillus species with pathogenic potential. Microbiology Spectrum. 2019;**2**:875-902. DOI: 10.1128/9781683670131.ch55

[11] Andersson A, Ronner U, Granum PE. What problems does the food industry have with the spore-forming pathogens *Bacillus cereus* and *Clostridium perfringens*? International Journal of Food Microbiology. 1995;**28**(1419):145-155

[12] Schoeni JL, Lee Wong AC. *Bacillus cereus* food poisoning and its toxins. Journal of Food Protection. 2005;**68**(3):636-648. DOI: 10.4315/0362-028X-68.3.636

[13] Haddaji N, Chakroun I, Fdhila K, Smati H, Bakhrouf A, Mzoughi R. Pathogenic impacts of *Bacillus cereus* strains on *Crassostrea gigas*. Foodborne Pathogens and Disease. 2022;**19**(2):1-8. DOI: 10.1089/fpd.2021.0050

[14] Hansen BM, Hendriksen NB. Detection of enterotoxic *Bacillus cereus* and *Bacillus thuringiensis* strains by PCR analysis. Applied and Environmental Microbiology. 2001;**67**(1):185-189. DOI: 10.1128/AEM.67.1.185

[15] Drobniewski FA. *Bacillus cereus* and related species. Clinical Microbiology

Reviews. 1993;**6**(4):324-338. DOI: 10.1128/CMR.6.4.324.Updated

[16] Forghani F, Kim JB, Oh DH. Enterotoxigenic profiling of emetic toxin- and enterotoxin-producing *Bacillus cereus*, isolated from food, environmental, and clinical samples by multiplex PCR. Journal of Food Science. 2014;**79**(11):M2288-M2293. DOI: 10.1111/1750-3841.12666

[17] Osimani A, Aquilanti L, Clementi F. *Bacillus cereus* foodborne outbreaks in mass catering. International Journal of Hospitality Management. 2018;**72**(May):145-153. DOI: 10.1016/j.ijhm.2018.01.013

[18] Ceuppens S, Boon N, Uyttendaele M. Diversity of *Bacillus cereus* group strains is reflected in their broad range of pathogenicity and diverse ecological lifestyles. FEMS Microbiology Ecology. 2013;**84**(3):433-450. DOI: 10.1111/1574-6941.12110

[19] Glasset B et al. *Bacillus cereus*-induced food-borne outbreaks in France, 2007 to 2014: Epidemiology and genetic characterisation. Euro Surveillance. 2016;**21**(48):1-11. DOI: 10.2807/1560-7917.ES.2016.21.48.30413

[20] Bennett SD, Walsh KA, Gould LH. Foodborne disease outbreaks caused by *Bacillus cereus*, *Clostridium perfringens*, and *Staphylococcus aureus*—United States, 1998-2008. Clinical Infectious Diseases. 2013;**57**(3):425-433. DOI: 10.1093/cid/cit244

[21] Rodrigo D, Rosell CM, Martinez A. Risk of *Bacillus cereus* in relation to rice and derivatives. Food. 2021;**10**(302):1-11. DOI: 10.3390/foods10020302

[22] Vilas-Bôas GT, Peruca APS, Arantes OMN. Biology and taxonomy of *Bacillus cereus*, *Bacillus anthracis*, and *Bacillus thuringiensis*. Canadian Journal of Microbiology. 2007;**53**(6):673-687. DOI: 10.1139/W07-029

[23] Food and Drug Administration. Bad Bug Book, Foodborne Pathogenic Microorganisms and Natural Toxins. Second ed. 2012. https://www.fda.gov/files/food/published/Bad-Bug-Book-2nd-Edition-%28PDF%29.pdf

[24] Haque MA, Quan H, Zuo Z, Khan A, Siddique N, He C. Pathogenicity of feed-borne *Bacillus cereus* and its implication on food safety. Agrobiological Records. 2021;**3**:1-16. DOI: 10.47278/journal.abr/2020.015

[25] Griffiths MW, Schraft H. *Bacillus cereus* Food Poisoning. Third ed. Elsevier Inc.; 2017. DOI: 10.1016/B978-0-12-385007-2.00020-6

[26] Kamar R et al. Pathogenic potential of *Bacillus cereus* strains as revealed by phenotypic analysis. Journal of Clinical Microbiology. 2013;**51**(1):320-323. DOI: 10.1128/JCM.02848-12

[27] Griffiths MW. *Bacillus cereus* and other *Bacillus* spp. Pathogens and Toxins in Foods: Challenges and Interventions. 2009:1-19. DOI: 10.1128/9781555815936.ch1

[28] Wijnands LM, Dufrenne JB, Rombouts FM, In't Veld PH, Van Leusden FM. Prevalence of potentially pathogenic *Bacillus cereus* in food commodities in the Netherlands. Journal of Food Protection. 2006;**69**(11):2587-2594. DOI: 10.4315/0362-028X-69.11.2587

[29] Granum PE et al. Evidence for a further enterotoxin complex produced by *Bacillus cereus*. FEMS Microbiology Letters. 1996;**141**(141):145-149. DOI: 10.1111/j.1574-6968.1996.tb08376.x

[30] Tewari A, Abdullah S. *Bacillus cereus* food poisoning: International and Indian perspective. Journal of Food Science and Technology. 2014;**52**(5):2500-2511. DOI: 10.1007/s13197-014-1344-4

[31] Lund T, De Buyser ML, Granum PE. A new cytotoxin from *Bacillus cereus* that may cause necrotic enteritis. Molecular Microbiology. 2000;**38**(2):254-261. DOI: 10.1046/j.1365-2958.2000.02147.x

[32] Ramm F, Stech M, Zemella A, Frentzel H, Kubick S. The pore-forming hemolysin bl enterotoxin from *Bacillus cereus*: Subunit interactions in cell-free systems. Toxins (Basel). 2021;**13**(807):1-17. DOI: 10.3390/toxins13110807

[33] Dietrich R, Jessberger N, Ehling-Schulz M, Märtlbauer E, Granum PE. The food poisoning toxins of *Bacillus cereus*. Toxins (Basel). 2021;**13**(2):1-48. DOI: 10.3390/toxins13020098

[34] Cufaoglu G, Ayaz ND. Potential risk of *Bacillus cereus* in spices in Turkey. Food Control. 2022;**132**:1-6. DOI: 10.1016/j.foodcont.2021.108570

[35] Melling J, Capel BJ, Turnbull PCB, Gilbert RJ. Identification of a novel enterotoxigenic activity associated with *Bacillus cereus*. Journal of Clinical Pathology. 1976;**29**(10):938-940. DOI: 10.1136/jcp.29.10.938

[36] Agata N, Ohta M, Mori M, Isobe M. A novel dodecadepsipeptide, cereulide, is an emetic toxin of *Bacillus cereus*. FEMS Microbiology Letters. 1995;**129**(1):17-19. DOI: 10.1111/j.1574-6968.1995.tb07550.x

[37] Walser V, Kranzler M, Ehling-Schulz M, Stark TD, Hofmann TF. Structure revision of isocereulide A, an isoform of the food poisoning emetic *Bacillus cereus* toxin cereulide. Molecules. 2021;**26**(5):1-12. DOI: 10.3390/molecules26051360

[38] Mahler H et al. Fulminant liver failure in association with the emetic toxin of *Bacillus cereus*. The New England Journal of Medicine. 1997;**336**(16):1142-1148. DOI: 10.1056/nejm199704173361604

[39] Agata N, Ohta M, Yokoyama K. Production of *Bacillus cereus* emetic toxin (cereulide) in various foods. International Journal of Food Microbiology. 2002;**73**(1):23-27. DOI: 10.1016/S0168-1605(01)00692-4

[40] Altayar M, Sutherland AD. *Bacillus cereus* is common in the environment but emetic toxin producing isolates are rare. Journal of Applied Microbiology. 2006;**100**(1):7-14. DOI: 10.1111/j.1365-2672.2005.02764.x

[41] Carlin F et al. Emetic toxin-producing strains of *Bacillus cereus* show distinct characteristics within the *Bacillus cereus* group. International Journal of Food Microbiology. 2006;**109**(1-2):132-138. DOI: 10.1016/j.ijfoodmicro.2006.01.022

[42] Agata N, Ohta M, Mori M. Production of an emetic toxin, cereulide, is associated with a specific class of *Bacillus cereus*. Current Microbiology. 1996;**33**(1):67-69. DOI: 10.1007/s002849900076

[43] Sastalla I et al. The *Bacillus cereus* Hbl and Nhe tripartite enterotoxin components assemble sequentially on the surface of target cells and are not interchangeable. PLoS One. 2013;**8**(10):1-13. DOI: 10.1371/journal.pone.0076955

[44] Schoeni JL, Lee Wong AC. Heterogeneity observed in the components of hemolysin BL, an enterotoxin produced by *Bacillus cereus*. International Journal of Food Microbiology. 1999;**53**(2-3):159-167. DOI: 10.1016/S0168-1605(99)00158-0

[45] Lund T, Granum PE. Characterisation of a non-haemolytic enterotoxin complex from *Bacillus cereus* isolated after a foodborne outbreak. FEMS Microbiology Letters. 1996;**141** (2-3):151-156. DOI: 10.1016/0378-1097 (96)00208-X

[46] Granum PE, O'Sullivan K, Lund T. The sequence of the non-haemolytic enterotoxin operon from *Bacillus cereus*. FEMS Microbiology Letters. 1999;**177**(2):225-229. DOI: 10.1016/ S0378-1097(99)00312-2

[47] Fagerlund A, Lindbäck T, Storset AK, Granum PE, Hardy SP. *Bacillus cereus* Nhe is a pore-forming toxin with structural and functional properties similar to the ClyA (HlyE, SheA) family of haemolysins, able to induce osmotic lysis in epithelia. Microbiology. 2008;**154**(3):693-704. DOI: 10.1099/ mic.0.2007/014134-0

[48] Castiaux V, Liu X, Delbrassinne L, Mahillon J. Is Cytotoxin K from *Bacillus cereus* a bona fide enterotoxin? International Journal of Food Microbiology. 2015;**211**:79-85. DOI: 10.1016/j.ijfoodmicro.2015.06.020

[49] Shadrin AM, Shapyrina EV, Siunov AV, Severinov KV, Solonin AS. *Bacillus cereus* pore-forming toxins hemolysin II and cytotoxin K: Polymorphism and distribution of genes among representatives of the cereus group. Microbiology. 2007;**76**(4):405-412. DOI: 10.1134/S0026261707040042

[50] Guinebretiere MH, Fagerlund A, Granum PE, Nguyen-The C. Rapid discrimination of cytK-1 and cytK-2 genes in *Bacillus cereus* strains bya novel duplex PCR system. FEMS Microbiology Letters. 2006;**259**(1):74-80. DOI: 10.1111/j.1574-6968.2006.00247.x

[51] Boonchai N, Asano SI, Bando H, Wiwat C. Study on cytotoxicity and nucleotide sequences of enterotoxin FM of *Bacillus cereus* isolated from various food sources. Journal of the Medical Association of Thailand. 2008;**91**(9):1425-1432

[52] Tran SL, Guillemet E, Gohar M, Lereclus D, Ramarao N. CwpFM (EntFM) is a *Bacillus cereus* potential cell wall peptidase implicated in adhesion, biofilm formation, and virulence. Journal of Bacteriology. 2010;**192**(10):2638-2642. DOI: 10.1128/JB.01315-09

[53] Hsieh YM, Sheu SJ, Chen YL, Tsen HY. Enterotoxigenic profiles and polymerase chain reaction detection of *Bacillus cereus* group cells and B. cereus strains from foods and food-borne outbreaks. Journal of Applied Microbiology. 1999;**87**(4):481-490. DOI: 10.1046/j.1365-2672.1999.00837.x

[54] Ngamwongsatit P et al. Broad distribution of enterotoxin genes (hblCDA, nheABC, cytK, and entFM) among *Bacillus thuringiensis* and *Bacillus cereus* as shown by novel primers. International Journal of Food Microbiology. 2008;**121**(3):352-356. DOI: 10.1016/j.ijfoodmicro.2007.11.013

[55] Granum PE. BACILLUS/ food poisoning. Encyclopedia of Food Sciences and Nutrition. 2003;7(1992):365-371. DOI: 10.1016/ b0-12-227055-x/00076-6

[56] Ramarao N, Lereclus D, Sorokin A. The *Bacillus cereus* Group. Vol. 2. Elsevier Ltd; 2015. DOI: 10.1016/ B978-0-12-397169-2.00059-7

[57] Beecher DJ, Wong ACL. Tripartite hemolysin BL from *Bacillus cereus*. Hemolytic analysis of component interactions and a model for its characteristic paradoxical zone phenomenon. The Journal of Biological

Chemistry. 1997;**272**(1):233-239. DOI: 10.1074/jbc.272.1.233

[58] FAO. The FAO Action Plan on Antimicrobial Resistance 2021-2025. Rome: FAO; 2021

[59] Fiedler G et al. Antibiotics resistance and toxin profiles of *Bacillus cereus*-group isolates from fresh vegetables from German retail markets. BMC Microbiology. 2019;**19**(1):1-13. DOI: 10.1186/s12866-019-1632-2

[60] Merzougui S, Lkhider M, Grosset N, Gautier M, Cohen N. Prevalence, PFGE typing, and antibiotic resistance of *Bacillus cereus* group isolated from food in Morocco. Foodborne Pathogens and Disease. 2014;**11**(2):145-149. DOI: 10.1089/fpd.2013.1615

[61] Chon JW, Kim JH, Lee SJ, Hyeon JY, Seo KH. Toxin profile, antibiotic resistance, and phenotypic and molecular characterization of *Bacillus cereus* in Sunsik. Food Microbiology. 2012;**32**(1):217-222. DOI: 10.1016/j.fm.2012.06.003

[62] Bernhard K, Schrempf H, Goebel W. Bacteriocin and antibiotic resistance plasmids in *Bacillus cereus* and *Bacillus subtilis*. Journal of Bacteriology. 1978;**133**(2):897-903. DOI: 10.1128/jb.133.2.897-903.1978

[63] Park YB et al. Prevalence, genetic diversity, and antibiotic susceptibility of *Bacillus cereus* strains isolated from rice and cereals collected in Korea. Journal of Food Protection. 2009;**72**(3):612-617. DOI: 10.4315/0362-028X-72.3.612

[64] Luna VA, King DS, Gulledge J, Cannons AC, Amuso PT, Cattani J. Susceptibility of *Bacillus anthracis*, *Bacillus cereus*, *Bacillus mycoides*, *Bacillus pseudomycoides* and *Bacillus thuringiensis* to 24 antimicrobials using Sensititre® automated microbroth dilution and Etest® agar gradient diffusion methods. The Journal of Antimicrobial Chemotherapy. 2007;**60**(3):555-567. DOI: 10.1093/jac/dkm213

[65] Citron DM, Appleman MD. In vitro activities of daptomycin, ciprofloxacin, and other antimicrobial agents against the cells and spores of clinical isolates of *Bacillus* species. Journal of Clinical Microbiology. 2006;**44**(10):3814-3818. DOI: 10.1128/JCM.00881-06

[66] Yu P et al. *Bacillus cereus* isolated from vegetables in China: Incidence, genetic diversity, virulence genes, and antimicrobial resistance. Frontiers in Microbiology. 2019;**10**(May):1-10. DOI: 10.3389/fmicb.2019.00948

[67] Lee N, Sun JM, Kwon KY, Kim HJ, Koo M, Chun HS. Genetic diversity, antimicrobial resistance, and toxigenic profiles of *Bacillus cereus* strains isolated from sunsik. Journal of Food Protection. 2012;**75**(2):225-230. DOI: 10.4315/0362-028X.JFP-11-317

[68] Owusu-Kwarteng J, Wuni A, Akabanda F, Tano-Debrah K, Jespersen L. Prevalence, virulence factor genes and antibiotic resistance of *Bacillus cereus* sensu lato isolated from dairy farms and traditional dairy products. BMC Microbiology. 2017;**17**(1):1-8. DOI: 10.1186/s12866-017-0975-9

[69] Arslan S, Eyi A, Küçüksari R. Toxigenic genes, spoilage potential, and antimicrobial resistance of *Bacillus cereus* group strains from ice cream. Anaerobe. 2014;**25**:42-46. DOI: 10.1016/j.anaerobe.2013.11.006

[70] Zhu L, He J, Cao X, Huang K, Luo Y, Xu W. Development of a double-antibody sandwich ELISA for rapid detection of *Bacillus cereus* in food. Scientific Reports. 2016;**6**:1-10. DOI: 10.1038/srep16092

[71] Vidic J, Chaix C, Manzano M, Heyndrickx M. Food sensing: Detection of *Bacillus cereus* spores in dairy products. Biosensors. 2020;**10**(3):1-16. DOI: 10.3390/bios10030015

[72] Andersson MA, Mikkola R, Helin J, Andersson MC, Salkinoja-Salonen M. A novel sensitive bioassay for detection of *Bacillus cereus* emetic toxin and related depsipeptide ionophores. Applied and Environmental Microbiology. 1998;**64**(4):1338-1343. DOI: 10.1128/aem.64.4.1338-1343.1998

[73] Chen G et al. Antibiotic-based magnetic Nanoprobes combined with mPCR for simultaneous detection of Staphylococcus aureus and *Bacillus cereus*. Food Analytical Methods. 2021;**14**(9):1964-1976. DOI: 10.1007/s12161-021-02026-z

[74] Wehrle E, Moravek M, Dietrich R, Bürk C, Didier A, Märtlbauer E. Comparison of multiplex PCR, enzyme immunoassay and cell culture methods for the detection of enterotoxinogenic *Bacillus cereus*. Journal of Microbiological Methods. 2009;**78**(3):265-270. DOI: 10.1016/j.mimet.2009.06.013

[75] Tawil N, Sacher E, Mandeville R, Meunier M. Bacteriophages: Biosensing tools for multi-drug resistant pathogens. Analyst. 2014;**139**(6):1224-1236. DOI: 10.1039/c3an01989f

[76] Schneider KR, Schneider RG, Silverberg R, Kurdmongkoltham P, Bertoldi B. Preventing foodborne illness: *Bacillus cereus*. EDIS. 2017;**14**:1-5

[77] Centers for Disease Control and Prevention (CDC). Surveillance for foodborne disease outbreaks—United States, 2015, Atlanta, Georg. US Department of Health and Human Services. CDC. 2017;**62**(1):1-24. DOI: 10.1016/j.annemergmed.2013.04.001

[78] Krishnamurthy K, Sneed J. Cooling practices used in school foodservice. Food Protection Trends. 2011;**31**(12):828-833

[79] Luu-Thi H et al. Carvacrol suppresses high pressure high temperature inactivation of *Bacillus cereus* spores. International Journal of Food Microbiology. 2014;**197**:1-38. DOI: 10.1016/j.ijfoodmicro.2014.12.016

[80] Ayari S, Dussault D, Hayouni EA, Hamdi M, Lacroix M. Radiation tolerance of *Bacillus cereus* pre-treated with carvacrol alone or in combination with nisin after exposure to single and multiple sub-lethal radiation treatment. Food Control. 2013;**32**:693-701. DOI: 10.1016/j.foodcont.2013.01.019

[81] Yang Y, Tao WY, Liu YJ, Zhu F. Inhibition of *Bacillus cereus* by lactic acid bacteria starter cultures in rice fermentation. Food Control. 2008;**19**:159-161. DOI: 10.1016/j.foodcont.2007.03.002

[82] Røssland E, Borge GIA, Langsrud T, Sørhaug T. Inhibition of *Bacillus cereus* by strains of *Lactobacillus* and *Lactococcus* in milk. International Journal of Food Microbiology. 2003;**89**:205-212. DOI: 10.1016/S0168-1605(03)00149-1

[83] Al-Qadiri HM et al. Bactericidal activity of neutral electrolyzed water against *Bacillus cereus* and *Clostridium perfringens* in cell suspensions and artificially inoculated onto the surface of selected fresh produce and polypropylene cutting boards. Food Control. 2019;**96**:212-218. DOI: 10.1016/j.foodcont.2018.09.019

[84] Henderson I, Duggleby CJ, Turnbull PCB. Differentiation of *Bacillus*

anthracis from other *Bacillus cereus* group bacteria with the PCR. International Journal of Systematic Bacteriology. 1994;**44**(1):99-105. DOI: 10.1099/00207713-44-1-99

[85] Manzano M, Cocolin L, Cantoni C, Comi G. *Bacillus cereus*, *Bacillus thuringiensis* and *Bacillus mycoides* differentiation using a PCR-RE technique. International Journal of Food Microbiology. 2003;**81**(3):249-254. DOI: 10.1016/S0168-1605(02)00222-2

Section 2

Foodborne Pathogen Dectection Methods

Chapter 4

Tools for Rapid Detection and Control of Foodborne Microbial Pathogens

Rajani Chowdary Akkina, Vijayalakshmi Payala and Sharon Sushma Maganti

Abstract

Foodborne illnesses have become more common over time, posing a major threat to human health around the world. Foodborne pathogens can be present in a variety of foods, and it is critical to detect them in order to ensure a safe food supply and prevent foodborne illnesses. Traditional methods for detecting foodborne pathogens are time-consuming and labor-intensive. As a result, a range of technologies for quick detection of foodborne pathogens have been developed, as it is necessary for many food analysis. Nucleic acid-based, biosensor-based, and immunological-based approaches are the three types of rapid detection methods. The ideas and use of modern quick technologies for the detection of foodborne bacterial infections are the focus of this chapter.

Keywords: foodborne illness, microorganisms, detection, traditional techniques, molecular methods

1. Introduction

Food poisoning, often known as foodborne illness, is caused by consuming infected food or beverages. Foodborne diseases are to blame for global morbidity and mortality. The gastrointestinal tract of the consumer is the primary organ affected by food infections, but few can target the neurological system, brain, or spinal cord. The researchers discovered more than 250 foodborne illnesses. During 2009–2015 Foodborne Disease Outbreak Surveillance System (FDOSS), received reports of 5760 outbreaks that resulted in 100,939 illnesses, 5699 hospitalizations, and 145 deaths in Columbia. Outbreaks caused by Listeria, Salmonella, and Shiga toxin-producing *Escherichia coli* (STEC) were responsible for 82% of all hospitalizations and 82% of deaths reported [1]. Food poisoning is usually caused by several forms of fungi, bacteria, viruses, and parasites. Food poisoning is thought to be caused by harmful toxins from both microbial and non-microbial sources. WHO estimates that in 2010, with a world population of 6.9 billion, global foodborne diseases resulted in 600 million illnesses, 420,000 deaths. Globally, animal-source foods—meats, fish, dairy products, and eggs—account for approximately one-third of the total burden of foodborne disease [2]. The rapid and precise monitoring and detection of foodborne pathogens are some of the most effective ways to control and prevent human foodborne infections. Traditional microbiological detection and identification methods for foodborne pathogens are well known to be time-consuming and laborious, as they are increasingly being perceived as insufficient to meet the demands of rapid food testing. Thus, there is a need for novel methods that can detect close to "real-time", small numbers of viable bacterial cells within a given volume of food. Recently, various kinds of rapid detection, identification, and monitoring methods have been developed for foodborne pathogens, including nucleic-acid-based methods, immunological methods, biosensor-based methods, etc. The application of biosensor technology offers promising solutions for portable, rapid, and sensitive detection of microorganisms in the food industry. To limit the spread of foodborne pathogens and outbreaks of foodborne illness, rapid, accurate, and reliable methods of identifying foodborne microbial pathogens are required [3].

1.1 Global burden of food borne disease

FBD is expected to cause 76 million illnesses, 325,000 hospitalizations, and 5000 fatalities in the United States per year, as well as 2,366,000 cases, 21,138 hospitalizations, and 718 deaths in England and Wales. Foodborne Disease Outbreak Surveillance System (FDOSS) received reports of 5760 outbreaks in Columbia between 2009 and 2015, resulting in 100,939 illnesses, 5699 hospitalizations, and 145 fatalities. Listeria, Salmonella, and Shiga toxin-producing *Escherichia coli* (STEC) outbreaks were responsible for 82 percent of all reported hospitalizations and deaths. With a global population of 6.9 billion people, WHO estimates that global foodborne infections caused 600 million illnesses and 420,000 deaths in 2010. Animal-source foods, such as meats, fish, dairy products, and eggs, account for almost one-third of the entire burden of foodborne disease worldwide (**Figure 1**) [2–6].

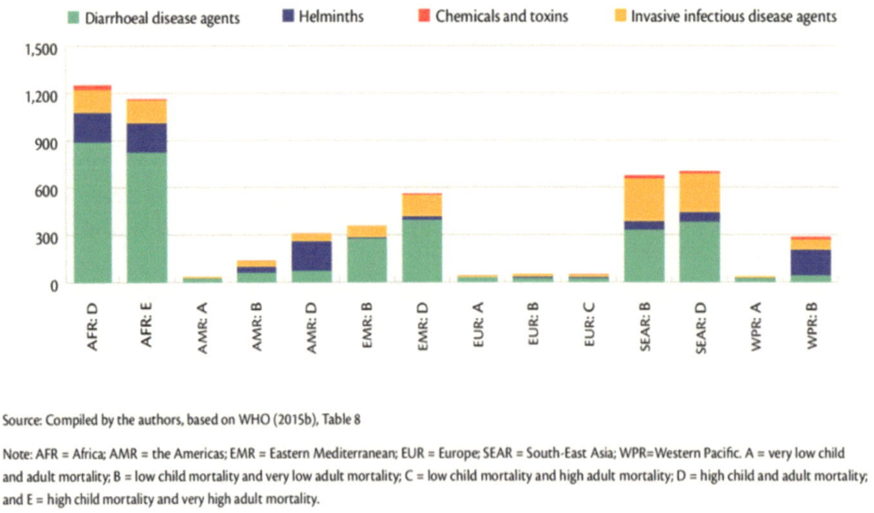

Figure 1.
The global burden of foodborne disease (DALYs per 100,000 population) by hazard groups and by subregion (Food systems and diets: Facing the challenges of the twenty first century, Lukasz Aleksandrowicz, Publisher: Global Panel on Agricultural and Food Systems for Nutrition).

2. Foodborne illness (causes and symptoms)

Food can be contaminated by infectious organisms or their poisons at any step during processing or manufacture. Food contamination can occur at any stage of production, including growing, harvesting, processing, storage, transporting, and preparation. Cross-contamination is a common cause, with hazardous organisms being transferred from one surface to another. Food poisoning can also be caused by eating raw or undercooked meat and poultry, seafood, or raw shellfish [7]. Nausea, vomiting, watery or bloody diarrhea, stomach pain and cramps, and fever are the most prevalent symptoms. The majority of symptoms are gastrointestinal, although they can also manifest as neurological, gynecological, malignant, and immunological disorders.

3. Pathogens causing foodborne illness

Foodborne pathogens are mainly bacteria, viruses, or even parasites that are present in the food and are the cause of major diseases such as food poisoning. **Table 1** showed the various common pathogens causing foodborne illness and its symptoms.

4. Detection methods

One of the most effective strategies to manage and prevent human foodborne diseases is to monitor and detect foodborne pathogens quickly and precisely. Traditional microbiological detection and identification procedures for foodborne pathogens are well known for being time-consuming and labor-intensive, and they are increasingly being seen as unable to fulfill the demands of rapid food testing. As a result, new approaches are needed to detect small quantities of viable bacterial cells in a given volume of food in near real-time. For foodborne pathogens, several types of quick detection, identification, and monitoring technologies, such as nucleic-acid-based methods, immunological methods, and biosensor-based methods, have recently been developed. Occasionally, false-negative or false-positive results are obtained, necessitating further investigation. ELISA is a very reliable and precise method for detecting a wide range of proteins in a complex matrix in both qualitative and quantitative terms. The use of biosensor technology in the food business offers promising solutions for portable, quick, and sensitive detection of microorganisms. The straightforward and easy-to-use immunomagnetic separation of *E. coli* O157:H7 employing aptamers-gold nanoparticle probe quenching Rhodamine B's fluorescence was performed. **Figure 2** showed the various detection methods of foodborne pathogens by conventional and novel strategies.

Food microbiological testing has always been an important aspect of the food production process, but it is most commonly used for end-product control. Microbiological testing has two main goals: determining the absence of pathogens or their toxins to ensure food safety, and determining the overall microbial load to determine product quality and shelf-life stability.

4.1 Traditional methods

Traditional culture methods cultivate, isolate, and enumerate the target microbe while simultaneously preventing the growth of other microorganisms contained in the

S. no.	Foodborne pathogens or their toxins	Predominant symptoms
1.	*Staphylococcus aureus* and its enterotoxins	Nausea, vomiting, retching, diarrhea, abdominal pain, prostration
2.	*Bacillus cereus* (emetic toxin)	Vomiting or diarrhea, depending on whether diarrheic or emetic toxin present; abdominal cramps; nausea
3.	Norovirus	Nausea, vomiting, watery non-bloody diarrhea, dehydration
4.	*Clostridium perfringens*	Abdominal cramps, diarrhea, putrefactive diarrhea (*C. perfringens*), sometimes nausea and vomiting
5.	*Salmonella* spp., *Shigella* spp., *E. coli*	Fever, abdominal cramps, diarrhea, vomiting, headache
6.	*Vibrio cholearae* (O1 and non-O1), *Vibrio parahaemolyticus*	Abdominal cramps, diarrhea, vomiting, fever, malaise, nausea, headache, dehydration
7.	Enterohaemorrhagic *E. coli*, *Campylobacter* spp.	Diarrhea (often bloody), abdominal pain, nausea, vomiting, malaise, fever (uncommon with *E. coli* O157:H7)
8.	Rotavirus, Astrovirus, enteric Adenovirus	Fever, vomiting, watery non-inflammatory diarrhea
9.	*Yersinia enterocolitica*	Fever, diarrhea, abdominal pain
10.	*Entamoeda histolytica*	Abdominal pain, diarrhea, constipation, headache, drowsiness, ulcers, variable—often asymptomatic
11.	*Taenia saginata*, *Taenia solium*	Nervousness, insomnia, hunger pains, anorexia, weight loss, abdominal pain, sometimes gastroenteritis
12.	*Clostridium botulinum* and its neurotoxins	Vertigo, double or blurred vision, loss or light reflex, difficulty in swallowing, dry mouth, weakness, respiratory paralysis
13.	*Trichinella spiralis*	Gastroenteritis, fever, edema around eyes, perspiration, muscular pain, chills, prostration, labored breathing
14.	*Salmonella tympi*	Malaise, headache, fever, fever, cough, nausea, vomiting, constipation, abdominal pain, chills, rose spots, bloody stools
15.	*Toxoplasma gondii*	Fever, headache, myalgia, rash
16.	*Listeria monocytogenes*, *Campylobacter jejuni*	Fever, chills, headache, arthralgia, prostration, malaise, swollen lymph nodes, and other specific symptoms of disease in question

Table 1.
Various microbial pathogens causing foodborne illness.

food using selective liquid or solid culture media. Pre-enrichment growth, selective enrichment culture, and selective plating are used to identify foodborne pathogens, followed by biochemical identification and serological confirmation of the results. Culture approaches are available in both qualitative and quantitative formats [8].

4.1.1 Culture-based methods

4.1.1.1 Qualitative

When only the presence or absence of a pathogen in a food sample must be determined, qualitative procedures are used, in which presumptive colonies are grown

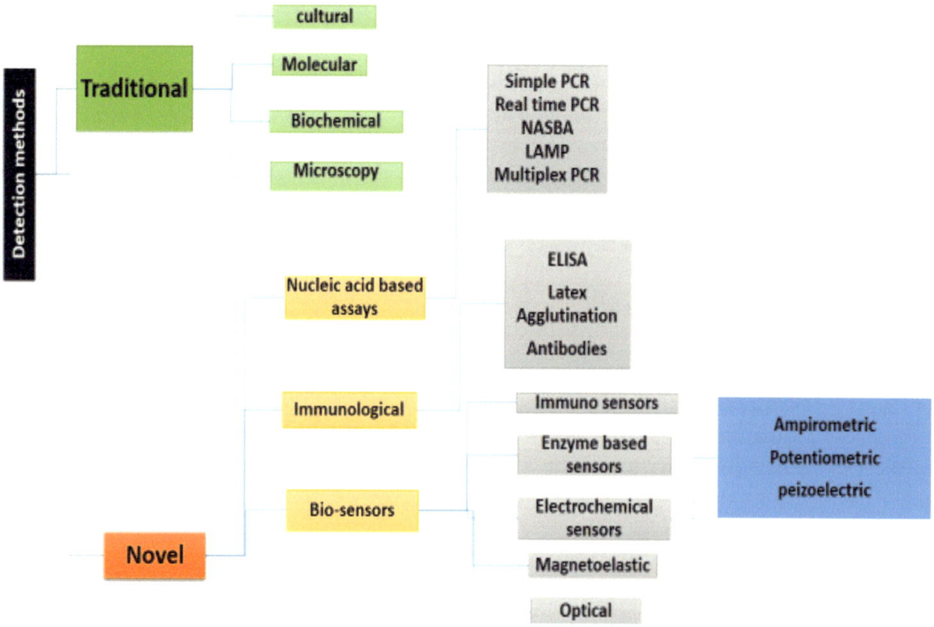

Figure 2.
Various detection methods of foodborne pathogens.

on selective media from a known amount of food. Pure cultures are raised, and the pathogen is identified using various biochemical or serological tests.

4.1.1.2 Quantitative

The plate count method or the most probable number method, both of which are based on serial dilution procedures, are used to count the microorganisms present in the food sample by culture method. Although these methods are reasonably affordable, sensitive, and still considered gold standards, their main disadvantage is their lengthy analysis time and labor-intensive nature. The entire operation usually takes between 7 and 10 days [9–11].

4.1.2 Microscope-based methods

Various approaches based on microscopic and optical traits of the suitably stained microbial cells have been developed for ensuring microbiological safety of foods and food products, these include:

4.1.2.1 Direct epifluorescent filter technique (DEFT)

It is a rapid way of enumerating microbial foodborne pathogens and is used commonly in the dairy sector for raw foods, milk and milk products, beverages, and snacks, among other things. Bacterial cells are captured on the surface of polycarbonate membrane filters, then stained with a fluorochrome like acridine orange and visualized using epifluorescence microscopy. The DEFT count is quick and precise, but it is very labor-intensive and is only useful when there are roughly 10^3 to 10^4 CFU/g of bacteria in the sample [12, 13].

4.1.2.2 Flow cytometry

It is applied to count the number of live bacteria in a sample and to analyze the viability, metabolic status, and antigenic markers of bacteria using fluorescent dyes. When cells are made to pass through a beam of light individually, this technique quantifies their optical properties. The procedure is quick, automatic, and specific if selectively discriminating dyes for specific species of bacteria are available. However, the detection limit for food samples is roughly10^5 to 10^7 CFU/g [13].

4.1.2.3 Solid phase cytometry (SPC)

The principles of epifluorescence microscopy and flow cytometry are combined in this method. Microorganisms are trapped on a membrane filter, fluorescently labeled, and counted automatically using a laser scanner. An epifluorescence microscope coupled to a scanning instrument by a computer-driven moving stage can visually inspect each fluorescent spot. SPC is appropriate only if the count of bacteria is around 10^3 to 10^4 CFU/g [13, 14].

4.1.3 Immunological methods

Antigen-antibody reactions underpin all immunological approaches for detecting foodborne infections. These responses are diverse and specific, but the immunoassay's success is determined by the antibody's specificity. With the emergence of hybridoma technology, monoclonal antibodies that specifically react just to one pathogen have been created. Immunoassays have a detection limit of approximately 10^4 to 10^5 CFU/g [13]. Immunoassays are offered in a variety of configurations.

4.1.3.1 Latex agglutination

Antibody-coated colored latex beads that agglutinate the target antigens (specific pathogen) and generate a visible precipitate are used to identify the food-borne pathogens. The latex agglutination assay is easy and quick, but it is not very sensitive and requires about 10^7 bacterial cells for the reaction to happen [15, 16].

4.1.3.2 Reverse passive latex agglutination test

Antibody-coated colored beads are used to agglutinate soluble antigens or toxins in place of microbiological cells to identify pathotoxins. The inert or carrier particle is attached to a known antibody rather than an antigen in this case. The active site of the antibody must be oriented to face outward. It's used to detect antigens from bacteria like Group A and B Streptococcus, *Mycoplasma pneumoniae*, *Staphylococcus aureus*, *Neisseria meningitides*, *Haemophilus influenza*, *Cryptococcus neoformans* [17, 18].

4.1.3.3 Immunodiffusion test

Antigen diffusion is allowed through an antibody-impregnated gel, and the formation of a precipitation line shows the presence of a certain foodborne pathogen or antigen.

4.1.3.4 Enzyme-linked immunosorbent assay (ELISA)

It is one of the most widely used and quick methods for detecting foodborne pathogenic bacteria. Most commercially available immunological kits use double antibody sandwich assays, which use commercially available antibody-coated microtiter plates (primary antibody) or other solid matrices to capture antigen (pathotoxin or pathogen) from target food samples, and then add a second antibody (secondary antibody) conjugated with an enzyme to form an antibody-antigen-conjugate "sandwich" [19].

4.2 Nucleic acid-based methods

These methods rely on the detection of certain gene sequences (signature sequences) in the target organism's genotype. The sequences can be chosen to detect a certain group, genus, species, or even strain of the microbe. There are many other types of DNA-based assays, but probes and nucleic acid amplification techniques are the most common and have been commercially developed for identifying foodborne infections.

4.2.1 Nucleic acid probes

Because probe-based tests are simple to apply, they are frequently employed in the food business. Nucleic acid probes are immobilized to inorganic substrates in these experiments so that they can be easily manipulated (e.g., washing out unhybridized DNA) without being damaged or lost. The use of DNA probes is based on a basic idea. It entails the use of a known DNA probe (labeled DNA) to hybridize the DNA sequence of an unknown microbial pathogen. Any microbial cells in the food sample that must be tested for pathogen presence are lysed, releasing their DNA, which is denatured, and the probe is added. The single-stranded DNA probe then hybridizes (annealing of complementary strands) with single-stranded DNA released from pathogenic bacteria present in the food. The signal is obtained by the hybridization of the labeled probe if the desired targeted sequence is present. The probe will not bind if the intended sequence is missing, and no signal will be obtained [15, 16].

4.2.2 Polymerase chain reaction (PCR)

PCR is currently a widely used and incredibly potent technology that allows for rapid exponential amplification of a specific target sequence, reducing the need for culture enrichment. With respect to a single pathogen in food, this approach can detect a single copy of a target DNA sequence. For the identification of microbial infections, PCR provides various benefits over culture and other traditional procedures, including sensitivity, specificity, accuracy, speed, and the ability to detect minute amounts of target nucleic acid in a sample. For the detection of food pathogens, PCR comes in a variety of formats [20, 21].

4.2.2.1 Ligase chain reaction PCR

LCR is a new technology that uses DNA amplification to detect the nucleic acid sequence of bacteria. It's comparable to PCR, except that only probe molecules amplify by nucleotide polymerization. To make a single probe, two probes for each DNA strand are ligated together. The reaction is driven by thermostable DNA polymerase and a DNA ligase enzyme in LCR. This method has one drawback in terms of food pathogen detection: it can detect DNA from dead species. It is one of the newest amplification approaches for finding point mutations in microbial pathogens. This method uses a thermostable ligase to distinguish between DNA sequences that differ only by a single base pair. LCR assay is commonly used for the specific recognition of *Listeria monocytogenes* [22].

4.2.2.2 Nucleic acid sequence-based amplification (NASBA)

NASBA was created primarily to detect RNA. It's a transcription-dependent amplification technique that uses promoter primers to recognize specific target sequences and synthesize RNA amplicons. Reverse transcriptase, Rnase H, and T7 RNA polymerase are three viral enzymes that work together to amplify RNA targets. A primer attaches to the target RNA sequence, and a reverse transcriptase produces a cDNA strand. The template RNA is subsequently digested by RNase H, and a second primer binds to cDNA, allowing the reverse transcriptase to generate double-stranded cDNA. Finally, T7 RNA polymerase is used in an amplification process to generate RNA transcripts. The main advantage of this approach is that it is isothermal, which eliminates the need for expensive thermal cyclers., NASBA diagnostics were originally developed for the identification of viruses, but they have also been used in food testing to detect *E. coli*, Campylobacter, *Salmonella enterica*, and *L. monocytogenes*, in a variety of foods, as well as *Cryptosporidium parvum* in water [23, 24].

4.2.2.3 Strand displacement amplification

Strand Displacement Amplification (SDA), is an isothermic amplification technique that uses four different primers, each with a Hind II exonuclease restriction site, DNA as a template, and an exonuclease-deficient fragment of *E. coli* DNA polymerase 1 (exo-Klenow) for primer elongation. About 10^9 copies of target DNA can be made in a single reaction. SDA is the basis for commercial detection assays like BD Probe Tec, and it has recently been tested for detecting *Mycobacterium tuberculosis* directly from clinical samples [25, 26].

4.2.2.4 Nested polymerase chain reaction

Nested polymerase chain reaction is a revision of polymerase chain reaction. Because it decreases non-specific binding in products caused by the amplification of unanticipated primer binding sites, this approach is more sensitive and specific than traditional PCR. Two sets of primers are utilized in two separate polymerase chain reaction runs in this procedure. The first set of primers is used to amplify a target sequence, which is subsequently employed as a template for a second amplification. The second primer set remains internal to the first amplicon. As a result, if the first amplification is nonspecific, secondary amplification does not occur. This innovative PCR approach has been used to detect a variety of foodborne pathogens, including *Vibrio parahaemolyticus*, *E. coli* O157:H7, Salmonella, *Listeria monocytogenes*, and *Staphylococcus aureus* [19]. NPCR was used to identify contamination of *Fusarium culmorum* in cereal samples [27].

4.2.2.5 Real-time PCR

Real-time polymerase chain reaction, also known as a quantitative real-time polymerase chain reaction, is a technique for amplifying and quantifying a specific DNA molecule in real-time. It has the ability to detect as well as quantify. The quantity can be either a perfect number of copies or a relative amount when normalized to DNA input or additional normalizing genes. The amplified DNA is detected in real-time as the process progresses. In real-time PCR, there are two main methods for detecting products: (1) non-specific fluorescent dyes, such as SYBR-green I, EtBr, and others, that intercalate with any double-stranded DNA. (2) Sequence-specific DNA probes, such as TaqMan, Molecular Beacons, Scorpions, and others, are comprised of oligonucleotides tagged with a fluorescent reporter that allows detection only after hybridization of the probe with its complementary DNA target. For the identification and characterization of food-borne diseases, a number of commercial kits based on real-time PCR technology are now available on the market [28–30].

4.2.2.6 Multiplex polymerase chain reaction

In the food industry, the expense and restricted volume of test samples are the most important factors to consider when evaluating quality. Multiple sets of primers are included in a single reaction tube in multiplex PCR, allowing more than one target sequence to be amplified in a single reaction system. A single test run can yield more information if numerous genes are targeted at the same time. The main benefit is that less reagent and enzyme (Taq DNA polymerase) are used. Another advantage is that, because pathogens are evaluated individually, sample preparation and findings are completed in a short amount of time. The only drawback is that amplified fragments of the same length cannot be distinguished, and a smaller amount of amplified product may not show up on an agarose gel. This could be solved by developing primers that are longer and have a higher melting temperature (Tm) than those used in conventional PCR [22, 24].

4.2.2.7 Low-stringency single-specific-primer PCR

Low-stringency Single-Specific-Primer PCR (LSSP-PCR) is a straightforward PCR technique for detecting single or multiple mutations in gene-sized DNA fragments. The first of the two steps are specific PCR (sPCR), which is used to obtain the DNA template, and the second is LSSP-PCR, which uses low-stringency conditions, and only one primer, which is commonly utilized in the sPCR. It's utilized to identify infectious pathogens like the Human Papilloma Virus (HPV), Trypanosoma cruzi, Trypanosoma rangeli, and Leishmania infantum by their genetic typing [30, 31].

4.2.2.8 Restriction fragment length polymorphism

Restriction Fragment Length Polymorphism (RFLP) is a very simple approach that involves the digestion of genomic DNA with certain restriction enzymes. It is used to compare the number and size (mass) of fragments produced by restriction endonucleases cutting at a certain recognition site of the target DNA molecule. Electrophoretic separation is used to examine the resultant DNA fragments. Presence, absence, or changes in the weight of the resultant DNA fragments are evidence of altering DNA sequences. For the species-level differentiation of bacteria, this approach requires pure culture. For the accurate detection of Staphylococcus and Listeria spp., RFLP in conjunction with PCR has been employed [32, 33].

4.2.2.9 Amplified fragment length polymorphism (AFLP)

Another genotyping approach is AFLP, which is based on the selective amplification of restriction segments of DNA molecules. The approach comprises digestion of whole pure genomic DNA using restriction endonucleases, followed by ligation of the resultant fragments with a double-stranded oligonucleotide adaptor complementary to the restriction site's base sequence. Primers corresponding to the contiguous base sequences in the adaptor, the restriction site, and one or more nucleotides in the original target DNA are used to selectively amplify sets of these fragments in PCR. Gel electrophoresis is used to examine the PCR-amplified DNA fragments. AFLP can be used to identify contamination sources, especially in cases involving live stocks [34, 35].

4.2.2.10 Random amplified polymorphic DNA technique

The Random Amplified Polymorphic DNA (RAPD) approach is a PCR experiment that can be used to distinguish races, strains, and pathogenic or non-pathogenic isolates using arbitrary primers. The primers used in this procedure are very short bits (10 or fewer bases) of DNA from a known source. It's very likely that these primers will be able to discover some complementary sequences in the target DNA, resulting in a variety of different-sized DNA fragments. When the results of such a reaction are studied using gel electrophoresis, various banding patterns emerge, some of which may be unique to certain species, varieties, or strains. Some pathogenic fungi may be detected and diagnosed using the patterns alone [36].

4.2.2.11 Loop-mediated isothermal amplification (LAMP)

The loop-mediated isothermal amplification (LAMP) approach for detecting target genes in food samples is a fast, accurate, and cost-effective method. Under isothermal circumstances, LAMP is a single-step amplification reaction that amplifies a target DNA sequence with high sensitivity and specificity. LAMP approach involves three phases, an initial phase, a cycling amplification step, and an elongation step. It uses a strand-displacement DNA polymerase, as well as two inner primers and two outer primers that recognize six different locations inside a target DNA. Because the amplification reaction happens only when all six areas inside a target DNA are appropriately recognized by the primers, the LAMP test is exceedingly specific. Visual judgment, rather than post-amplification electrophoresis, simplifies detection. LAMP has been used to detect a variety of pathogens that cause foodborne illnesses. LAMP kits have been commercially produced for detecting Legionella, Salmonella, Campylobacter Listeria, and verotoxin-producing *Escherichia coli* [37, 38].

4.2.2.12 Repetitive extragenic palindromic PCR

Because of the many typing methods employed in terms of time, accuracy, and cost, rep-PCR may be able to obtain rapid, accurate, and higher resolution findings among the various strains involved in the hospital outbreak. REP PCR was recently utilized in Italy to identify and classify *Ochrobactrum anthropi* strains. During their hospitalization at Catanzaro University Hospital (Italy) Oncology O.U Institution, all of the patients became infected. There had never been any cases of *O. anthropi* infection before. This was a more precise, efficient, and strong tool for bacterial typing and monitoring, as well as nosocomial infection control [39, 40].

4.2.2.13 DNase treated DNA (DTD) PCR

The key benefit of this technology is that it avoids the issues that PCR-based techniques have with the quick detection of foodborne pathogens. The challenge of testing a single organism at a time was solved by using a multiplex PCR approach. To discover a solution to the problem of false-positive results acquired by amplification of DNA from dead cells, DNase I enzyme treatment followed by PCR (that is DTD-PCR) was tried. When the multiplex procedure was examined for specificity, no interferences or non-specific amplification were identified. As a result, this DTD multiplex PCR technique may be practically used to identify viable cells of four major pathogens, including *Listeria monocytogenes*, *E. coli* O157:H7, *Salmonella enterica*, and *Vibrio parahaemolyticus* [41].

4.3 Nanoparticles in pathogen detection

The manipulation of matter on an atomic, molecular, and supramolecular scale is known as nanotechnology ("nanotech"). Bacteria, poisons, proteins, and nucleic acids can now be bound to these nanoparticles thanks to advancements in nanomaterial manipulation. One of the most significant advantages of employing nanomaterials for bio-sensing is their enormous surface area, which allows a greater number of biomolecules to be immobilized, increasing the number of reaction sites accessible for interaction with a target species. This characteristic, in combination with strong electrical and optical properties, makes nanomaterials ideal for "label-free" detection and the development of biosensors with higher sensitivity and faster response times. AuNPs (gold nanoparticles) have been employed in a variety of optical and electrical tests. Gold nanoparticles (AuNPs) have been employed in a variety of optical and electrical assays because of their high conductivity. *Salmonella typhimurium* and *E. coli* O157:H7 organisms are detected with AuNPs at concentrations of 98.9 cfu/mL and 1–10 cfu/mL, respectively. Quantum dots (2–10 nm) made up of semiconducting fluorescent nanoparticles with a semiconductor material core (often cadmium combined with selenium or tellurium) and an additional semiconductor shell (typically zinc sulfide) detected *E. coli* 0157:H7 10^3 cfu/ml (brain, heart infusion broth). Multi-walled nanotubes (MWNTs, 2–100 nm) are simply a number of concentric single-walled nanotubes (SWNTs, 0.4–3 nm) that exhibit photoluminescence and have good electrical properties; semiconductors are employed for the detection of *E. coli* O157:H7 at the 1 cell/mL limit. The detection of dsDNA and ssDNA was attempted using non-functional AuNPs. Citrate-coated AuNPs in this approach has a distinctive red color in the colloidal state. The addition of salts can easily cause AuNPs to aggregate, resulting in a purple color; the change in color can be seen with the naked eye. The negatively charged AuNPs interact electrostatically with ssDNA, which can uncoil in such a way that its hydrophilic negatively charged phosphate backbone is exposed to aqueous solutions, and DNA bases interact with the AuNPs surface via VanderWaals forces, giving the AuNPs a negative charge and increasing their repulsion. These characteristics have been used to create a biosensor that can detect a PCR product in the same tube within minutes. In comparison to existing approaches, the created biosensor is very selective and sensitive, and it can detect low levels of DNA [42–44].

4.4 Biosensors

Pathogenic microbes have been found in common foods such as milk, cheese, pork, chicken, raw vegetables, and fruits. The pathogens can be determined using standard procedures in about 1–2 days. Biosensors are the most promising new tool for combating this problem. A biosensor is an analytical instrument that translates biological signals and responses into electrical signals. This comprises two key components: a bioreceptor that recognizes the event and a transducer that converts the recognition event into a quantifiable sensitive electrical signal. A bioreceptor can be a microbe, organelle, cell, tissue, antibody, enzyme, nucleic acid, biomimic, or a combination of the above, and the transduction can be thermometric, electrochemical, optical, piezoelectric, or magnetic.

4.4.1 Immunosensors

Biosensors based on the interactions of specific antibodies with a specific antigen are known as immunosensors. Antigens detect antibody binding by immobilizing the reaction on the surface of a transducer, which translates surface change parameters into detectable electrical impulses. Bioreceptors can be monoclonal, polyclonal, or recombinant, depending on their qualities and the method they are synthesized. In eggs and chicken meat, a sandwich immunoassay was developed for two Salmonella species (*S. gallinarum* and *S. pullorum*). According to the researchers, a linear response to Salmonella species was found in the concentration range of 10^4 to 10^9 CFU/ mL, and the detection limit for both species was 3.0 10^3 CFU/mL. Xu et al. investigated immunosensors functioning with screen-printed interdigitated microelectrode (SP-IDME) transducers [39]. The immunosensor was capable of identifying E. coli O157:H7 and *S. typhimurium* in pure culture samples at concentrations of 10^2 to 10^6 CFU/mL, according to their findings. For the detection of *S. typhimurium* in milk, a cadmium selective polymeric membrane microelectrode (Cd-ISE) was used as a transducer. The detection limit was discovered to be 2 cells per 100 μL. In their study, they found that the average total time per assay for detecting *S. typhimurium* in milk samples was 75 minutes [45–47].

4.4.2 Enzyme-based biosensors

On fluorescent and radiolabeled compounds, enzyme as a bio receptor provides a number of advantages. The enzyme immunoassay reagents are non-hazardous, stable, and sensitive. By immobilization, the enzyme bio receptor is properly linked to the transducer. Enzymes are chosen based on their unique binding capabilities and catalytic activity, as well as a suitable substrate that allows for enough electron transport to the working. Storage stability, sensitivity, high selectivity, short reaction time, and great reproducibility are all advantages of enzyme immobilization. By labeling the antibody with enzymes, pathogenic bacteria such as *L. monocytogenes*, *E. coli*, and *C. jejuni* can be detected. Horseradish peroxidase (HRP) and beta-galactosidase are the most often used enzymes [48].

4.4.3 Electrochemical biosensors

Biosensors that measure electrochemical responses are known as electrochemical biosensors. They convert the incoming electrical signal directly into an electronic field, allowing small system designs with simple instrumentation to be created. Electrochemical biosensors are categorized as impedimetric, potentiometric, amperometric, and conductometric biosensors. For the detection of *S. aureus*, a simple label-free electrochemiluminescence (ECL) biosensor was created. In that investigation, the ECL intensity declined linearly with *S. aureus* concentrations ranging from 1.0×10^3 to 1.0×10^9 CFU/mL, with a detection limit of 3.1×10^2 CFU/mL. According to the author when a ready-to-use biosensor was used, the entire experiment could be completed in 70 minutes [49].

4.4.4 Amperometric biosensors

Electrochemical processes are studied using amperometric biosensors, which measure current changes in a constant potential. The biosensors' reaction is proportional to the concentration of analyte in a solution. Amperometric biosensors can be set up using two or three electrodes. The researchers developed an amperometric immunosensor for detecting *S. aureus* in food samples. The increase in amperometric response was used to measure the alterations. For *S. typhimurium* detection in milk, an amperometric biosensor was used, which demonstrated qualitative behavior with a very low limit of detection of 101 CFU/mL and a detection time of 125 minutes.

4.4.5 Potentiometric biosensors

Potentiometric biosensors rely on the detection of oxidation and reduction potential of an electrochemical reaction. As a result, a pH meter comprises an immobilized enzyme membrane around the probe, where the catalyzed process produces or absorbs hydrogen ions. Ion-selective electrodes are used in potentiometric biosensors to turn the biological reaction into an electrical signal. Potentiometric biosensors detect potential changes below zero degrees Celsius. Field-effect transistor (FET) devices are used in recent potentiometric devices. Potentiometric biosensors based on carbon nanotubes and aptamers were used to detect *E. coli*, *S. aureus*, and *S. epidermidis* in pigskin, with a working range of 2.4×10^3 to 2.0×10^4 CFU/mL [50]. Piezoelectric biosensors, which work on the idea of directly detecting bacteria without the need for labeling, are fascinating sensors. In general, the bacteria-containing solution is deposited on the surface of the piezoelectric sensor, which is coated with a selective binding agent (e.g. antibodies). As the crystal mass increases, bacteria bind to antibodies, lowering the oscillation frequency. The pathogen (*S. aureus*) was detected in culture and milk using a piezoelectric biosensor, and the results ranged between 4.1×10^1 and 4.1×10^5 CFU/mL [51].

4.4.6 Magnetoelastic biosensors

Magnetoelastic sensors are constructed with amorphous ferromagnetic alloys. Remote sensing is a feature of magnetoelastic sensors, as the signal transmission takes place at a distance from the coil. The materials display a magnetoelastic resonance when triggered by a changing magnetic field, which may be detected using a noncontact signal collection coil. When a target comes into contact with the pathogen alloy sensor surface, the extra mass creates a shift in the resonance frequency, which the signal collector coil can detect from a distance. Magnetoelastic sensors, as a result, are wireless devices that can be highly useful for remote monitoring. The first wireless biosensors in biosensor platforms are magnetoelastic biosensors. A magnetoelastic biosensor with a working range of 5×10^1 to 5×10^8 CFU/mL was used to detect *S. typhimurium* on the tomato surface [52].

4.5 Pulse field gel electrophoresis

PFGE (Pulse Field Gel Electrophoresis) employs restriction enzymes, which are molecular scissors that cut bacterial DNA at probable restriction sites. These molecular scissors create a DNA imprint that is segregated by size. The bacteria are first placed in an agarose slurry, which is comparable to gelatin, and then the bacterial cell is opened to allow the DNA to be released. Listeria, Salmonella, *E. coli*, and other food-borne pathogens have all been identified using PFGE [45].

4.5.1 Multi locus enzyme electrophoresis (MLEE)

MLST and Multi Locus Enzyme Electrophoresis (MLEE) are useful for determining population structures of non-bacterial haploid infectious agents and for portable molecular typing of those agents that are weakly or strongly cloned. MLEE is commonly used for typing and population genetic analysis of pathogenic fungi and parasites. MLST is a nucleotide-based typing approach that determines a sequence type by analyzing data from housekeeping genes. MLST provides highly selective molecular typing data that can be electronically transferred between laboratories, making it ideal for studying the genetic relationship of bacteria. Some significant pathogens, such as *Haemophilus influenzae*, *Streptococcus pneumoniae*, and *Neisseria meningitides*, have been tested with the approach [53, 54].

4.6 Ribotyping

Ribotyping is a DNA-based subtyping procedure in which restriction enzymes are used to break bacterial DNA into fragments. The restriction enzymes utilized include PFGE, which cut DNA into larger pieces, although genomic DNA is cut into a large number of smaller fragments ranging from 1 to 30 kb in size in the ribotyping assay. Electrophoresis is used to separate the pieces according to their size. Furthermore, in southern blotting, DNA probes are selectively bound to target DNA containing genes coding for rRNA synthesis and are hybridized (to probe specific) for the 16S to 23S rRNA genes. For the distinction of *L. monocytogenes* and the characterization of virulence gene polymorphism lineages, automated ribotyping was used [46].

4.7 Plasmid profile analysis

The examination of plasmid DNA profiles has been utilized to type a variety of gram-negative and gram-positive bacteria. In the sphere of health care, it is applied and employed as a marker for comparing strains and assessing the potential spread of a resistance gene. Plasmids are unique in that they can be transferred to another strain by conjugation under selection pressure, but they can also be gained or lost spontaneously during the process. The acquisition or deletion of plasmid causes genetic relatedness to the isolate to become muddled, limiting short-term epidemiological research. This is particularly beneficial for species such as Staphylococcus spp. and enterobacteria [47].

4.8 Lipidomics

Lipidomics is an emerging active topic of biomedical and molecular research that involves complex lipidome analysis. Lipidome is a quantitative and complete description of a total lipid moiety present in an organism. Thousands of networks in different species, as well as their interactions with other lipids, carbohydrates, proteins, and other moieties, are identified and quantified in vivo. Membrane-lipidomics (description of membrane lipid constituents) and mediator-lipidomics (description of low abundance bioactive lipid constituents) are two subtypes of lipidomics. The study of pathogen lipid profiles is not entirely new. Liquid chromatography and mass spectrometry are driving the study of lipidomics, allowing for the perception, characterization, and quantification of a wide range of lipid classes. Capturing the entire "lipidome" of a cell or tissue in a single experiment is a difficult endeavor. The research will pave the door for the discovery of pathogen-specific metabolic pathways. Cell and molecular biology will be used as a unique way to analyze the intricate lipid signaling during host-pathogen interactions for medication and biomarker development [55].

5. Conclusions

Traditional methods for detecting foodborne pathogens, which rely on culturing methods, are efficient and gold standard methods but time-consuming and labor-intensive. As a result, a variety of quick detection approaches like PCR, application microarray technology, biosensors, etc. have been developed to address the limitations of traditional detection methods. To avoid outbreaks of foodborne diseases and the transmission of foodborne pathogens, quick methods for detecting foodborne pathogens in food products are critical. Traditional methods are less sensitive, specific, time-efficient, labor-saving, and dependable than rapid detection approaches.

Conflict of interest

Nil.

Author details

Rajani Chowdary Akkina[1*], Vijayalakshmi Payala[2] and Sharon Sushma Maganti[1]

1 Department of Microbiology and Food science and Technology, GITAM Institute of Science, GITAM, Deemed to be University, Visakhapatnam, Andhra Pradesh, India

2 Department of Microbiology, GITAM Institute of Medical Sciences and Research, GITAM, Deemed to be University, Visakhapatnam, Andhra Pradesh, India

*Address all correspondence to: rajaniagis@gmail.com

IntechOpen

© 2022 The Author(s). Licensee IntechOpen. This chapter is distributed under the terms of the Creative Commons Attribution License (http://creativecommons.org/licenses/by/3.0), which permits unrestricted use, distribution, and reproduction in any medium, provided the original work is properly cited.

References

[1] U.S. Food and Drug Administration. Foodborne illness: What you need to know. 2018. Available from: https://www.fda.gov/food/resourcesforyou/consumers/ucm103263.htm [Accessed: April 4, 2019]

[2] Li M, Havelaar AH, Hoffmann S, Hald T, Kirk MD, Torgerson PR, et al. Global disease burden of pathogens in animal source foods, 2010. PLoS One. 2019;**14**(6):e0216545

[3] Senturk E, Aktop S, Sanlibaba P, Tezel BU. Biosensors: A novel approach to detect food-borne pathogens. Applied Microbiology. Open Access. 2018;**4**:1-8

[4] Todd EC. Worldwide surveillance of foodborne disease: The need to improve. Journal of Food Protection. 1996;**59**(1):82-92

[5] Lynch MJ, Leon-Velarde CG, McEwen S, Odumeru JA. Evaluation of an automated immunomagnetic separation method for the rapid detection of Salmonella species in poultry environmental samples. Journal of Microbiological Methods. 2004;**58**(2):285-288

[6] Lian F, Wang D, Yao S, Ge L, Wang Y, Zhao Y, et al. A detection method of *Escherichia coli* O157: H7 based on immunomagnetic separation and aptamers-gold nanoparticle probe quenching Rhodamine B's fluorescence. Food Science and Biotechnology. 2021;**30**(8):1129-1138

[7] Centers for Disease Control and Prevention. Foodborne Germs and Illnesses. Centers for Disease Control and Prevention. Atlant. 2020

[8] Jasson V, Jacxsens L, Luning P, Rajkovic A, Uyttendaele M. Alternative microbial methods: An overview and selection criteria. Food Microbiology. 2010;**27**(6):710-730

[9] Betts R, de Blackburn CW. Detecting pathogens in food. In: Foodborne Pathogens. Cambridge: Woodhead Publishing; 2009. pp. 17-65

[10] Blodgett R, Food and Drug Administration. Bacteriological Analytical Manual. Appendix 2 Most Probable Number from Serial Dilutions. Food and Drug Administration; 2010. Available from: https://www.fda.gov/Food/FoodScienseResearch/LaboratoryMethods/ucm109656.htm

[11] Biswas AK. Evaluation of export buffalo meat for some chemical residues and microbial contaminants [Doctoral dissertation]. Izatnagar: Indian Veterinary Research Institute; 2005

[12] Hermida M, Taboada M, Menéndez S, Rodríguez-Otero JL. Semi-automated direct epifluorescent filter technique for total bacterial count in raw milk. Journal of AOAC International. 2000;**83**(6):1345-1348

[13] López-Campos G, Martínez-Suárez JV, Aguado-Urda M, López-Alonso V. Microarray Detection and Characterization of Bacterial Foodborne Pathogens. Springer Science & Business Media; 2012

[14] D'Haese E, Nelis HJ. Rapid detection of single cell bacteria as a novel approach in food microbiology. Journal of AOAC International. 2002;**85**(4):979-983

[15] Feng P. Impact of molecular biology on the detection of foodborne pathogens. Molecular Biotechnology. 1997;7(3):267

[16] Glynn B, Lahiff S, Wernecke M, Barry T, Smith TJ, Maher M. Current and emerging molecular diagnostic technologies applicable to bacterial food safety. International Journal of Dairy Technology. 2006;**59**(2):126-139

[17] Terry Kotria. 2. Basic Immunology Procedure. Austin Community College; 2010. Available from: www.austincc.edu/kotrla/SerLec2.pdf

[18] Mangal M, Bansal S, Sharma SK, Gupta RK. Molecular detection of foodborne pathogens: A rapid and accurate answer to food safety. Critical Reviews in Food Science and Nutrition. 2016;**56**(9):1568-1584

[19] Wiedmann M, Wilson WJ, Czajka J, Luo J, Barany F, Batt CA. Ligase chain reaction (LCR)-overview and applications. PCR Methods and Applications. 1994;**3**(4):S51-S64

[20] Rossen L, Nørskov P, Holmstrøm K, Rasmussen OF. Inhibition of PCR by components of food samples, microbial diagnostic assays and DNA-extraction solutions. International Journal of Food Microbiology. 1992;**17**(1):37-45

[21] Cook N. The use of NASBA for the detection of microbial pathogens in food and environmental samples. Journal of Microbiological Methods. 2003;**53**(2):165-174

[22] Min J, Baeumner AJ. Highly sensitive and specific detection of viable *Escherichia coli* in drinking water. Analytical Biochemistry. 2002;**303**(2):186-193

[23] Anthony RM, Brown TJ, French GL. Rapid diagnosis of bacteremia by universal amplification of 23S ribosomal DNA followed by hybridization to an oligonucleotide array. Journal of Clinical Microbiology. 2000;**38**(2):781-788

[24] Kawasaki S, Fratamico PM, Kamisaki-Horikoshi N, Okada Y, Takeshita K, Sameshima T, et al. Development of the multiplex PCR detection kit for Salmonella spp., *Listeria monocytogenes*, and *Escherichia coli* O157: H7. Japan Agricultural Research Quarterly: JARQ. 2011;**45**(1):77-81

[25] Kim JS, Lee GG, Park JS, Jung YH, Kwak HS, Kim SB, et al. A novel multiplex PCR assay for rapid and simultaneous detection of five pathogenic bacteria: *Escherichia coli* O157: H7, Salmonella, *Staphylococcus aureus*, *Listeria monocytogenes*, and *Vibrio parahaemolyticus*. Journal of Food Protection. 2007;**70**(7):1656-1662

[26] Klemsdal SS, Elen O. Development of a highly sensitive nested-PCR method using a single closed tube for detection of *Fusarium culmorum* in cereal samples. Letters in applied Microbiology. 2006;**42**(5):544-548

[27] Abravaya K, Huff J, Marshall R, Merchant B, Mullen C, Schneider G, Robinson J. Molecular beacons as diagnostic tools: Technology and applications. Clinical Chemistry and Laboratory Medicine. 2003;**41**(4):468-474

[28] Shi XM, Long F, Suo B. Molecular methods for the detection and characterization of foodborne pathogens. Pure and Applied Chemistry. 2010;**82**(1):69-79

[29] Wang K, Tang Z, Yang CJ, et al. Molecular engineering of DNA: Molecular beacons. Angewandte Chemie International edition in English. 2009;**48**(5):856-870

[30] Alvarenga JS, Ligeiro CM, Gontijo CM, Cortes S, Campino L, Vago AR, Melo MN. KDNA genetic signatures obtained by LSSP-PCR

analysis of Leishmania (Leishmania) infantum isolated from the new and the old world. PLoS One. 2012;7(8):e43363

[31] Vago AR, Macedo AM, Oliveira RP, Andrade LO, Chiari E, Galvao LM, et al. Kinetoplast DNA signatures of *Trypanosoma cruzi* strains obtained directly from infected tissues. The American Journal of Pathology. 1996;**149**(6):2153

[32] Paillard D, Dubois V, Duran R, Nathier F, Guittet C, Caumette P, et al. Rapid identification of Listeria species by using restriction fragment length polymorphism of PCR-amplified 23S rRNA gene fragments. Applied and Environmental Microbiology. 2003;**69**(11):6386-6392

[33] Ueda F, Anahara R, Yamada F, Mochizuki M, Ochiai Y, Hondo R. Discrimination of *Listeria monocytogenes* contaminated commercial Japanese meats. International Journal of Food Microbiology. 2005;**105**(3):455-462

[34] Siemer BL, Nielsen EM, On SL. Identification and molecular epidemiology of *Campylobacter coli* isolates from human gastroenteritis, food, and animal sources by amplified fragment length polymorphism analysis and Penner serotyping. Applied and Environmental Microbiology. 2005;**71**(4):1953-1958

[35] Lima CS, Pfenning LH, Costa SS, Campos MA, Leslie JF. A new Fusarium lineage within the *Gibberella fujikuroi* species complex is the main causal agent of mango malformation disease in Brazil. Plant Pathology. 2009;**58**(1):33-42

[36] Williams JG, Kubelik AR, Livak KJ, Rafalski JA, Tingey SV. DNA polymorphisms amplified by arbitrary primers are useful as genetic markers. Nucleic Acids Research. 1990;**18**(22):6531-6535

[37] Song T, Toma C, Nakasone N, Iwanaga M. Sensitive and rapid detection of Shigella and enteroinvasive *Escherichia coli* by a loop-mediated isothermal amplification method. FEMS Microbiology Letters. 2005;**243**(1):259-263

[38] Mori Y, Notomi T. Loop-mediated isothermal amplification (LAMP): A rapid, accurate, and cost-effective diagnostic method for infectious diseases. Journal of Infection and Chemotherapy. 2009;**15**(2):62-69

[39] Quirino A, Pulcrano G, Rametti L, Puccio R, Marascio N, Catania MR, et al. Typing of *Ochrobactrum anthropi* clinical isolates using automated repetitive extragenic palindromic-polymerase chain reaction DNA fingerprinting and matrix-assisted laser desorption/ionization–time-of-flight mass spectrometry. BMC Microbiology. 2014;**14**(1):1-8

[40] Bathe S, Achouak W, Hartmann A, Heulin T, Schloter M, Lebuhn M. Genetic and phenotypic microdiversity of Ochrobactrum spp. FEMS Microbiology Ecology. 2006;**56**(2):272-280

[41] NaNadugala LM, Rakshit SK. DNase treated DNA multiplex polymerase chain reaction assay for rapid detection of viable food borne pathogens. Journal of the National Science Foundation of Sri Lanka. 2009;**35**(4):1-9

[42] Yang L, Bashir R. Electrical/electrochemical impedance for rapid detection of foodborne pathogenic bacteria. Biotechnology Advances. 2008;**26**(2):135-150

[43] Wang C, Irudayaraj J. Gold nanorod probes for the detection of multiple pathogens. Small. 2008;**4**(12):2204-2208

[44] Rho S, Kim SJ, Lee SC, Chang JH, Kang HG, Choi J. Colorimetric detection

of ssDNA in a solution. Current Applied Physics. 2009;**9**(2):534-537

[45] Xu M, Wang R, Li Y. Rapid detection of *Escherichia coli* O157: H7 and *Salmonella typhimurium* in foods using an electrochemical immunosensor based on screen-printed interdigitated microelectrode and immunomagnetic separation. Talanta. 2016;**148**:200-208

[46] Fei J, Dou W, Zhao G. A sandwich electrochemical immunosensor for *Salmonella pullorum* and *Salmonella gallinarum* based on a screen-printed carbon electrode modified with an ionic liquid and electrodeposited gold nanoparticles. Microchimica Acta. 2015;**182**(13):2267-2275

[47] Zhao X, Lin CW, Wang J, Oh DH. Advances in rapid detection methods for foodborne pathogens. Journal of Microbiology and Biotechnology. 2014;**24**(3):297-312

[48] Sharma H, Agarwal M, Goswami M, Sharma A, Roy SK, Rai R, et al. Biosensors: Tool for food borne pathogen detection. Veterinary World. 2013;**6**(12):968

[49] Yue H, Zhou Y, Wang P, Wang X, Wang Z, Wang L, et al. A facile label-free electrochemiluminescent biosensor for specific detection of *Staphylococcus aureus* utilizing the binding between immunoglobulin G and protein A. Talanta. 2016;**153**:401-406

[50] Zelada-Guillén GA, Sebastián-Avila JL, Blondeau P, Riu J, Rius FX. Label-free detection of Staphylococcus aureus in skin using real-time potentiometric biosensors based on carbon nanotubes and aptamers. Biosensors and Bioelectronics. 2012;**31**(1):226-232

[51] Lian Y, He F, Wang H, Tong F. A new aptamer/graphene interdigitated gold electrode piezoelectric sensor for rapid and specific detection of *Staphylococcus aureus*. Biosensors and Bioelectronics. 2015;**65**:314-319

[52] Li S, Li Y, Chen H, Horikawa S, Shen W, Simonian A, et al. Direct detection of *Salmonella typhimurium* on fresh produce using phage-based magnetoelastic biosensors. Biosensors and Bioelectronics. 2010;**26**(4):1313-1319

[53] Jefferies J, Clarke SC, Diggle MA, Smith A, Dowson C, Mitchell T. Automated pneumococcal MLST using liquid-handling robotics and a capillary DNA sequencer. Molecular Biotechnology. 2003;**24**(3):303-307

[54] Romano S, Aujoulat F, Jumas-Bilak E, Masnou A, Jeannot JL, Falsen E, et al. Multilocus sequence typing supports the hypothesis that *Ochrobactrum* anthropi displays a human-associated subpopulation. BMC Microbiology. 2009;**9**(1):1-8

[55] Wenk MR. Lipidomics of host–pathogen interactions. FEBS Letters. 2006;**580**(23):5541-5551

Chapter 5

Advances in the Bacteriophage-Based Precise Identification and Magnetic Relaxation Switch Sensor for Rapid Detection of Foodborne Pathogens

Yiping Chen, Junping Wen, Junpeng Zhao and Chenxi Huang

Abstract

The development of novel and highly specific technologies for the rapid and sensitive detection of foodborne pathogens is very important for disease prevention and control. Bacteriophages can recognize viable and unviable bacteria, replacing antibodies as the recognition element in the immune response, which are currently being widely developed in novel precise identification biosensors. Magnetic relaxation switch sensors based on the magnetic relaxation signal has been used to construct a variety of background-free novel biosensors in recent years, which can realize rapid detection of foodborne pathogens. This chapter will mainly introduce the latest developments and future prospects of bacteriophages in the field of accurate identifications for foodborne pathogens. At the same time, it will introduce the research progress and development direction of novel magnetic relaxation switch sensors for detecting foodborne pathogens.

Keywords: foodborne pathogens, bacteriophage-based precise identification, magnetic relaxation switch sensors

1. Introduction

Food safety is one of the key issues that people are most concerned about. Food poisoning caused by foodborne diseases is a major problem in food safety. Pathogens are infectious agents that can cause foodborne diseases, which include fungi, protozoans, bacteria and viruses. They enter the human body through various modes of infection like food, water and air, and are responsible for deaths worldwide. The major foodborne pathogens include *Salmonella*, *Listeria monocytogenes*, *Escherichia coli*, *Campylobacter*, and *Staphylococcus aureus*. These pathogens are ubiquitous, which not only affect the quality of food ingredients, destroy nutritional components, but also can induce different diseases in humans by directly invasion or secreting certain toxins, leading to serious health risks and economic burdens [1]. Pathogen diagnosis

IntechOpen

requires convenient and rapid analytical methods to provide accurate identification. Highly sensitive and accurate analytical methods are also essential for timely clinical decision-making and management of epidemics for infectious diseases [2]. Meanwhile, identifying pathogens rapidly in the early stage of infection is significant to decrease high mortality caused by ingestion of contaminated foods [3].

Biosensors are a high-tech analytical device developed by the interdisciplinary integration of physics, chemistry and biology. They mainly use biomolecular recognition elements (such as antibodies, enzymes, nucleic acids, etc.) to recognize the targets analyte, and then converts to optical, electrical, magnetic or other signals that are easy to capture and recognize by a transducer for easy readout. Because of its advantages of high efficiency, easy automation and simple operation, it has been widely used in the field of food safety [4, 5].

It is anticipated that the future research direction of developing novel biosensors is to achieve the accurate identification of pathogens and eliminate the interference from food sample impurities. As emerging technologies, bacteriophage can recognize viable and unviable pathogens and can be a precise recognition element to replace traditional antibodies in the immune response, contributed to construct various precise biosensors. And the magnetic relaxation switch sensors which can realize high signal-to-noise ratio and background-free detection have also attracted extensive attention in the field of rapid detection for foodborne pathogens. In recent years, extraordinary progress has been made in terms of bacteriophage- and biosensor-based detection methods, focusing on their potential use in the field of rapid detection for foodborne pathogens, and becoming frontier research hotspot. This chapter will mainly introduce the latest developments and future prospects of bacteriophage-based precise identification technologies, which allow accurate detection of foodborne pathogens. Additionally, it will summarize the research progresses and development directions of novel magnetic relaxation switch sensors in the field of rapid detection for foodborne pathogens.

2. Introduction of bacteriophage

Bacteriophages (shortened to phage), composed of protein and nucleic acid, are viruses that can specifically infect bacteria and proliferate in host bacteria. Phage was first discovered by Frederick W. Twort in 1915 and subsequently isolated by Felixd'Herelle in 1917, who named phages according to their properties [6]. According to their basic structural forms, phages can be classified into icosahedral phages without tail structure, icosahedral phages with tail structure, and filamentous phages. Most phages are icosahedral phages with tail structure [7]. The head capsid and tail are composed of proteins. These phages consist of thehead capsids containing the genetic material of the phage (DNA or RNA), and the tails that have special receptors to recognize the cell surface of the host bacteria, which are related to phage specificity (**Figure 1**). Phage typically could also be categorized into lytic or temperate phages based in their life cycle.

Especially in the recent years, with a better understanding of the detailed knowledge phage characteristics, its application in clinical disease treatment, foodborne pathogen detection and other aspects has been gradually expanded. Phages offer several advantages, such as simple structure, easy to generate quantities in within a short time, high specificity to host bacteria, harmless to human, good stability, and the ability to distinguish viable and unviable bacteria. Their short preparation time

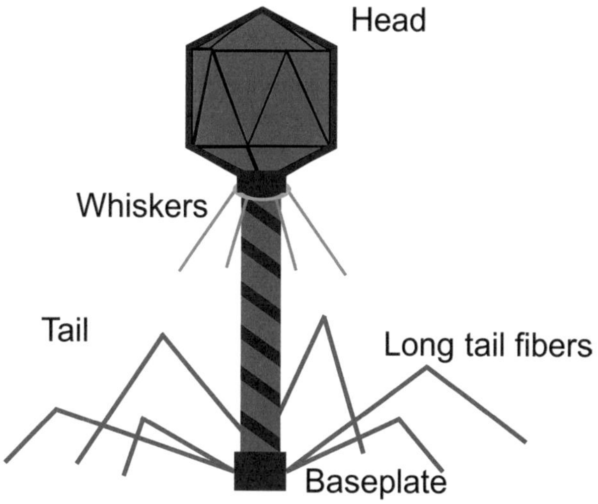

Figure 1.
Structure of a typical bacteriophage.

and low cost are also the advantages over antibodies. Based on these advantages, a variety of methods have been developed to detect pathogenic bacteria that using phages as the probes. Phages have shown a good application prospect in the field of rapid detection for pathogenic bacteria.

Compared with biometric elements such as antibodies and nucleic acids, phages have obvious advantages in the detection of pathogenic bacteria [8]. The features of bacteria and phages including specific interactions between phages and target bacterial cells, their infectious ability and phage-induced cell lysis, provide a basis for the detection of pathogenic bacteria [9]. At present, the phage-based detection methods are mainly based on phages (natural phages or recombinant phages) and phage components as recognition elements. Phage-based detection methods mainly include phage amplification, phage-based biosensors which combined natural phages with biosensors (such as electrochemistry biosensors and optics biosensors) and engineered phage-based methods (such as reporter phages and phage display technology). Phage component-based assays are mainly conducted by taking advantage of phage receptor binding proteins and lysin proteins. This part will discuss the research progress of the current phage-based detection methods to provide a comprehensive theoretical basis for food safety assessment.

2.1 Progress in detection methods using phage as recognition element

2.1.1 Phage amplification

Phage amplification is a classical method for the detection of foodborne pathogens. The principle of this strategy was based on the measurement of progeny phage released from the infected target bacteria. Specifically, phages were mixed with the sample solution to infect the target bacteria. Then the viricides such as ammonium ferrous sulfate are used to kill the free phages in the culture medium. After phages were released from the lysed target bacteria, the helper bacteria cells were added to propagate the phages and determine the phage titer using the double-layer plate method, so as to evaluate the number of target bacteria. This method has been used for the detection of *Mycobacterium tuberculosis*, *Salmonella*, *Listeria monocytogenes*, *Escherichia coli*, *Pseudomonas aeruginosa* and *Campylobacter* [10].

Rajnovic et al. developed a method based on the analysis of optical density kinetics in bacterial cultures with lysed MS2 phage for bacterial infection. This method can detect as few as 10 phage particles per assay volume after a phage incubation period of 3.5 h. And it could detect as low as 10^4 CFU/mL *Escherichia coli* in 2 h [11]. Garrido-Maestu et al. developed a novel method based on the amplification of the *Salmonella* bacteriophage vB_SenS_PVPSE2, coupled with real-time PCR (qPCR) for the rapid detection of viable *Salmonella* Enteritidis in chicken samples [12].

2.1.2 Phage-mediated biosensors

Phage-mediated biosensors can be divided into two categories in principle. One is to use phages as recognition and capture components of pathogenic bacteria, supplemented by other substances for signal readout, but it donot lyse bacteria. The other is to use naturally occurring lytic phages to specifically lyse host bacteria and release intracellular substances, which in turn trigger the catalysis of the substances to produce signals for readout. In this section, we will review the recent developments of these two detection methods.

Due to their advantages of high sensitivity, specificity, accuracy, fast response and low cost, sensors have become one of the most widely used methods in the detection of pathogenic bacteria. Zhou et al. developed a carbon nanotube (CNT)-based impedimetric biosensing method for rapid and selective detection of viable *Escherichia coli* B cells. The T2 bacteriophage (virus) served as the biorecognition element, which was immobilized on polyethylenimine (PEI)-functionalized carbon nanotube transducer on glassy carbon electrode. The detection was highly selective toward the B strain of *Escherichia coli* and the detection limit of the biosensor is 10 CFU/mL [13]. In a recent study, Farooq et al. isolated *Staphylococcus aureus*-specific phages and immobilized them on modified bacterial cellulose/carboxylated multiwalled carbon nanotubes to create an electrochemical biosensor to detect bacteria in milk samples. Results showed that 3 CFU/mL bacteria were detected in the phosphate buffer and 5 CFU/mL bacteria could be detected in the milk sample within 30 min at neutral pH [14]. Optical sensor is also one of the sensors that has been widely used in detecting pathogenic bacteria. Edgar et al. constructed the detection method of *Escherichia coli* by combining Quantum dot and phage for the first time in 2006. Tawil et al. developed a biosensor using whole phage and surface plasmon resonance to detect methicillin-resistant *Staphylococcus aureus* (MRSA) at 10^3 CFU/mL [15].

Phages are used to specifically lyse host bacteria to release intracellular enzymes or other specific substances. The released enzymes act as markers to catalyze the reaction of active substances to produce specific substances and generate signals that can be measured by biosensors, so as to detect pathogenic bacteria [16]. The intracellular enzymes that can be used as markers mainly include adenylate kinase, β-D-galactosidase, β-D-glucuronidase, etc. Chen et al. immobilized T7 phage particles on magnetic beads to capture and lyse *Escherichia coli* BL12, and then to release intracellular β-galactosidase (**Figure 2**). The detection limit within 2.5 h was about 1×10^4 CFU/mL, and it was reduced to 10 CFU/mL after 6 h pre-enrichment [17].

In addition, researchers combined phages and bioluminescence reagents to develop optical-based methods, such as ATP bioluminescence, NADH bioluminescence for pathogenic bacteria detection. First of all, the target bacteria were

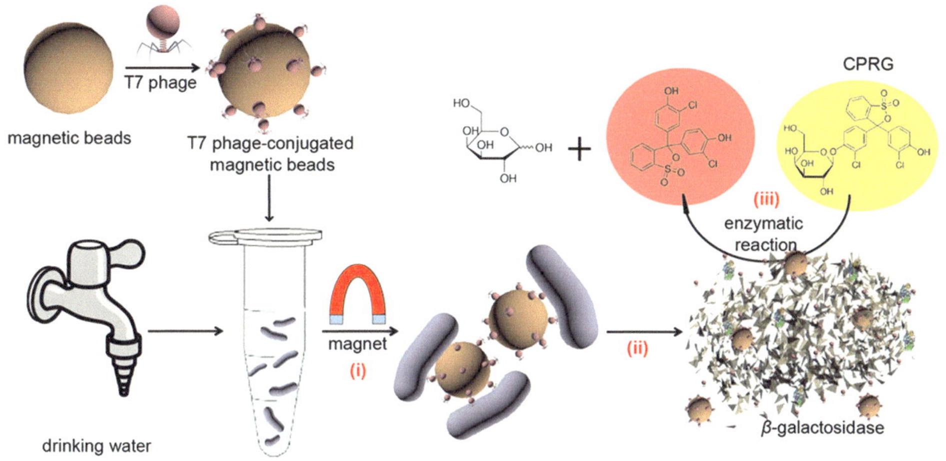

Figure 2.
Schematic representation of detection of Escherichia coli *in drinking water using T7 bacteriophage-conjugated magnetic probe [17]. Copyright 2015 American Chemical Society.*

subjected to phage specific infection, and lysed to release ATP and NADH, since the content of ATP and NADH in each cell was roughly constant. ATP is then catalyzed by luciferase to react with luciferin or NADH with substrates such as FMN and aldehydes to emit light [18]. Bacterial count could be evaluated from quantitative measurements of ATP bioluminescence. Eed et al. developed an ATP bioluminescence-sensing assay to detect microbial viability. A bioluminescent recombinant *Escherichia coli* strain was used with luciferase extracted from transformed bacteria. Results showed that this method were more rapid and efficient than traditional plate counting assay [19].

2.1.3 Progress in detection methods based on engineered phage

Reporter phage detection techniques are based on molecular biology methods. In this method, the reporter phage containing the reporter gene is constructed first. The reporter gene is introduced into the host chromosome and encodes the expression of a fluorescent substance or a colorimetric marker dependent substrate for pathogen identification.

Reporter genes commonly used at present include firefly luciferase gene (luc), bacterial luciferase gene *(luxAB)* [20], green fluorescent protein gene (*gfp*), bacterial ice nucleoprotein gene (*inaW*) [21] and β-D-galactosidase gene (*lacZ*) [22]. The proteins expressed by these genes in target bacteria can be detected using colorimetry, fluorescence or luminescence techniques. Reporter phage technology has been successfully used to identify a variety of pathogens, including *Escherichia coli*, *Mycobacterium*, *Salmonella*, *Staphylococcus aureus*, *Listeria monocytogenes*. The greatest advantage of reporter phage is its ability to distinguish between viable and unviable bacteria, since phage will not be able to infect and express reporter genes in unviable bacteria. Alcaine et al. constructed a lateral flow detection method for pathogenic bacteria by bioengineering T7 phage. This assay can detect 10^3 CFU/mL of *Escherichia coli* in broth after 7 h [23].

Phages have the unique ability to display peptides or proteins on their surfaces and can be used for the detection of foodborne pathogens. This technique named as phage display as first discovered in 1985. The proteins or peptides displayed are capable of affiniting to a variety of targets such as carbohydrates, proteins, small molecules, or whole cells. The basic principle is to fuse the gene encoding for the target peptide or proteinto the phage surface protein encoding gene, causing the mixed protein to be expressed on the phage surface [24]. Bacteriophage (M13, F1, FD, T4 and T7, etc.) are commenly used in phage display technology. McIvor et al. panned out *Listeria monocytogenes* polypeptides from the phage display peptide library with the ability to distinguish *Listeria monocytogenes* from other *Listeria* spp., which may have potential utility to enhance detection of *Listeria monocytogenes* [25]. Karoonuthaisirit et al. screened peptides specific to 8 *Salmonella* mixtures from the phage display peptide library. Meanwhile, SPR was used to detect *Salmonella* based on the screened phage polypeptides, and was capable of detection with high specificity and accuracy. The detection limits of 8.0×10^7 and 1.3×10^7 CFU/mL for one-time and five-time immobilized sensors, respectively [26].

2.2 Progress in detection methods using phage components

Phage components, such as RBP and lysins, not only have specific affinity to target bacteria, but also are highly adaptable to environmental conditions. RBP, located in the tail of the virion, anchor the phage to the host cell during infection by recognizing unique protein or carbohydrate (polysaccharide) sequences on the surface of the host bacteria [27]. Lysins are phage-encoded enzymes produced in infected host bacteria at the end of the lytic cycle. These hydrolases enable the phage to lyse the host cell from within and the release of progeny phage particles.

The RBP of phage not only has unique host tail recognition specificity that can specifically recognize host bacteria, but also hashigh resistance to environmental conditions, such as pH, temperature and resistance stability. The RBP of phage can be used as a potential probing element for pathogen detection. Singh et al. reported the use of the RBP of *Campylobacter* bacteriophage NCTC 12673 for the specific capture of *Campylobacter jejuni* bacteria using RBP-derivatized capturing surfaces. The detection limit of the RBP-derivatized SPR surfaces was found to be 10^2 CFU/mL [28]. Poshtiban et al. attached phage RBP Gp047 of phage NCTC12673 to magnetic beads. The specificity of capture was confirmed by using *Salmonella* Typhimurium as negative control. Total sample preparation and analysis time were less than 3 hours [29]. The specific RBP was displayed in engineered M13 phage, which has a natural potency to target the desired bacteria. The phages were bound on gold nanoparticles due to the available thiolation potency. The interaction was monitored through SPR, which detected 100 cells of *Escherichia coli* in less than 60 min [30].

Tolba et al. used the anchor region of *Listeria* bacteriophage produced lysin on the bacterial cell wall as the detection matrix to measure the change of electrochemical impedance during sample passage with a limit of detection limit as 10^5 CFU /mL in milk [31]. Chibli et al. exploited the ability of specific phage proteins, the endolysins LysK and Φ11, and the bacteriocin lysostaphin, fixed on silicon wafers to bind staphylococci. Binding was quantified by clearing assays in solution and by functionalization of silicon wafers followed by light microscopy. Bacterial binding densities on functionalized surfaces were ~3 cells/100 μm^2 [32]. Brzozowsk et al. presented a new type of highly sensitive label-free sensor based on long-period gratings (LPG) coated with T4 bacteriophage (phage) adhesin. The adhesin (gp37) binds *Escherichia coli* B by recognizing its bacterial lipopolysaccharide (LPS) [33]. The application of phage for pathogenic bacteria detection have been summary in **Table 1**.

In general, the mechanism of phage's specific adsorption on host bacteria, the advantages of phage and its application in the detection of pathogenic bacteria are introduced in this part. Phage has great application potential in the detection of pathogenic bacteria due to its advantages of good stability, easy preparation, strong specificity, high safety, and ability to distinguish viable and unviable bacteria. Bacteriophage component-based assays may have some advantages over the use of full phage particles. Phage proteins exhibit greater stability to extreme pH and temperature. The smaller protein size allows for more intensive surface modifications and targeted chemical functionalization to enhance the binding activity of these surfaces compared to the whole phage. In some cases of applications, phage-derived proteins offer another advantages, including captured intact bacteria without inducing lysis and releasing toxic products. The application of phage-derived proteins, while promising to replace antibodies used to capture and enrich bacterial pathogens, is still in its infancy and its potential is largely untapped.

In addition to the wide application of phage-based accurate identification in the field of food safety, the development of effective novel biosensing technologies with low background has also shown great application prospects. Nowadays, the application of magnetic relaxation switch (MRS) sensors in the rapid detection of foodborne pathogens increasingly attracted attention. Compared to traditional optical signal, the magnetic signal owns high specificity, for which the signal is negligible especially in biological and environmental samples. The developing MRS assays do not require complex separation and purification steps and can be performed in turbid, opaque and non-uniform medium, enabling background-free detection [34, 35]. Besides, the MRS senosrs have the advantages of fast detection, simple operation, high signal-to-noise ratio, and easy to realize on-site detection, which holds great promise for food safety. Based on this, we reviewed the MRS sensors research progress in the field of rapid detection for foodborne pathogens in next part.

Target	Limit of detection	Method	References
Escherichia coli	10^4 CFU/mL	Phage amplification	[11]
Salmonella	8 CFU /25 g		[12]
Escherichia coli	10 CFU/mL	Biosensor	[13]
Staphylococcus aureus	3 CFU/mL		[14]
Escherichia coli	10^3 CFU/mL		[15]
Escherichia coli	10^4 CFU/mL		[17]
Escherichia coli	10^3 CFU/mL	Engineered phage	[23]
Salmonella	1.3×10^7 CFU/mL	Phage display	[26]
Campylobacter jejuni	10^2 CFU/mL	Phage components	[28]
Escherichia coli	100 cells		[30]
Listeria	10^5 CFU /mL		[31]
Staphylococci	3 cells/100 μm^2		[32]

Table 1.
Application of phage in detection of pathogenic bacteria.

3. Introduction of magnetic relaxation switch sensors

Magnetic relaxation switch sensor has been an up-and-coming biosensing technology in recent years. It uses magnetic relaxation time as a signal readout to qualitatively and quantitatively detect targets. In physics, the relaxation refers to the process of returning to an equilibrium state after a certain equilibrium state is destroyed. Classical MRS sensors generally uses magnetic material as signal probe for detection. The magnetic nanoparticles (MNPs) are a kind of promising materials that can be extensively explored in various fields including clinical medicine, magnetic resonance imaging, data storage and food safety due to their unique size and physicochemical properties [36]. The basic principle of MRS sensors is the shortening of the relaxation time of water molecules mediated by MNPs, which can result in the nonuniform magnetic field. We can measure relaxation time of water protons through the process of relaxation, and relaxation time can be used as signal readout to reflect the amounts of targets. The relaxation time includes longitudinal relaxation time (T_1) and transverse relaxation time (T_2). In recent years, with the in-depth study of MNPs and relaxation mechanism, a series of magnetic sensors have been designed and worked at the molecular and cellular levels that combine with relaxation time as signal readout for target detection [37, 38].

Conventional MRS assay is generally based on the aggregation or dispersion of nanoparticles leading to the change of relaxation signal, as shown in **Figure 3** [39]. The application of MRS sensor started in 2001 by Weissleders's group, who use four different types of molecular interactions (DNA-DNA, protein-protein, protein-small molecule and enzyme catalysis) to show that the nanoparticles MRS technology can detect targets in vivo with highsensitivity, efficiency, and high-throughput. This platform is based the functional superparamagnetic nanoparticles (SMNPs) aggregated or dispersed *via* the specific affinity reaction between antibodies and antigens, and the quantity of target analyte was closely related to the degree of the state change, associated with a considerable change of the T_2 [35]. This research lay an important foundation of MRS sensor that particularly used to analyze various biochemical samples, such as nucleic acids, pathogens, biomacromolecules and micromolecules by inducing the aggregation or dispersion of MNPs and then bringing about a switch of the relaxation time to reflect the amounts of targets. The following part will summarize the research progress of MRS sensors following classification of state-dependent MRS sensors, amount-dependent MRS sensors, paramagnetic-ion mediated MRS sensors and other MRS sensors.

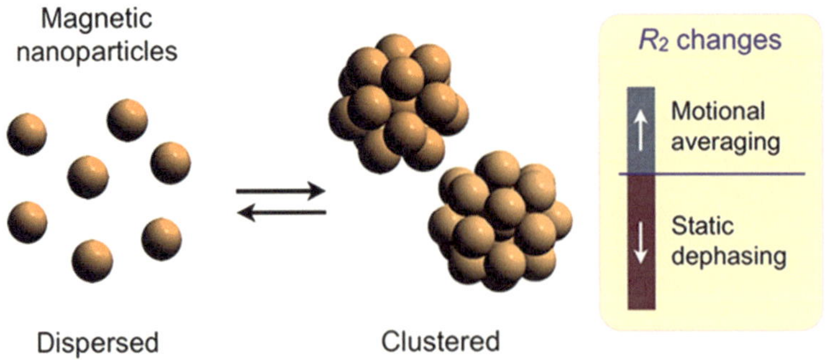

Figure 3.
The principle of classic magnetic relaxation switch (MRS) sensors [39]. Copyright 2012 American Chemical Society.

3.1 State-dependent MRS sensors for pathogens detection

The principle of MRS sensors based on magnetic particles changed state is to modify the donor/receptor (such as antigen/antibody, biotin/streptavidin, aptamers, etc.) on the surface of magnetic particles to construct specific magnetic probe. In the process of analysis, the specific recognition of the donor-receptor causes the state to change from dispersion to aggregation, hence affected the uniformity of the local magnetic field. When the water molecules diffuse through these uneven magnetic fields, the lateral relaxation of protons is accelerated and caused shorter lateral relaxation time [40]. The degree of magnetic probe state and T_2 signal change are positively correlated with the content of the target substance in the sample, so as to achieve the purpose of quantitative detection.

Based on this principle, Zhao et al. proposed a sensitive and rapid method for detecting *Listeria monocytogenes* (*L. monocytogenes*) in food which is based on the change of T_2 using NMR. Firstly, nanoparticles modified with silica and coupled with anti-*L. monocytogenes* antibodies dispersed in solution. Once the target of *L. monocytogenes*was added in solution, the functioned particles self-assembled on the surface of *L. monocytogenes* bring about the increase of the T_2 value of water protons. This method has a lower limit of detection limit of 3 MPN (using the most-probable-number (MPN) assay) and the upper limit of 10^3 CFU/mL and only requires 40 min to complete all the tests [41]. Based on a similar principle, Yu et al. developed a reliable immunoassay for the specific detection of *Cronobacter sakazakii* in dairy samples with silica-coated magnetic particles to ensure the safety of infant formula powder. This method is able to detect *Cronobacter sakazakii* in milk powder and cheese samples at 1.1–11 MPN, but does not fit for the detection of bacteria at higher concentrations (>1100 MPN) [42].

Except through the change of T_2 to judge result, Wang et al. developed a MRS sensor based on SMNPs which uses T_2 for signal readout for the rapid detection of the foodborne pathogen *Salmonella* in milk samples directly. The SMNPs can switch their dispersion and aggregation states based on the presence or absence of the target, which can adjust the T_2 of adjacent water molecules. Before the immune response, the state of SMNPs was dispersed, and the value of T_2 was high. After recognition by the immune response, SMNPs changed from dispersed to clustered, and the T_2 decreased rapidly. The value was positively correlated with the concentration of *Salmonella*, thus realizing the detection of *Salmonella* in milk samples. Compared with traditional ELISA, the sensitivity of this immunosensor is increased by 20 times (MRS, 10^3 CFU/mL; ELISA, 2×10^4 CFU/mL), and the required detection time is drastically reduced from 2 to 4 h to 30 min [43]. Apart from these pathogens, *Mycobacterium avium* spp. *Paratuberculosis* (MAP) is the known pathogen of Johne's disease in cattle, which is an economically devastating disease. This bacteria is difficult to grow in culture and its identification with current methods are difficult. Except causing severe intestinal inflammation in cattle, this microorganism has been isolated from blood, breast milk, and intestinal lesions of human patients. Kaittanis et al. realized the detection *of* MAP in milk using MRS sensor. The scheme is based on disperse nanoparticles in solution that can capture to the surface of a bacterial molecular and induce significant changes in T_2. As the amounts of bacteria increases, the available nanoparticles in solution were in a more disperse-like state, causing minimal changes in T_2. The detection limit is 1.55×10^3 CFU/mL, and the detection process was only 30 min without interference from other bacteria [44]. Subsequently, the same group reported the use of hybridizing magnetic nanosensors (hMRS) for the detection of MAP within less than an hour. The hMRS are designed to bind to a unique genomic sequence found in the MAP genome, causing significant changes in the sample's magnetic resonance signal. Hence they realized the detection of pathogens which can evade recognition by the immune system. This platform can detect a single MAP genome copy within 30 min [45].

Sara et al. proposed NMR-based detection system to detect pathogenic levels of *Vibrio parahaemolyticus* isolated from seafood with molecular mirroring using iron nanoparticles coated with target-specific biomarkers capable of binding to DNA of the target microorganism. The detection limit was 10^{5} CFU/mL, and was used to prevent the pathogen spread into humans, *via* contaminated, raw, or undercooked seafood [46]. A high affinity and specificity of the aptamer-recognition system was established by Jia's group that the anti-*Pseudomonas aeruginosa* (*P. aeruginosa*) aptamer was immobilized onto the surface of superparamagnetic iron oxide. Then the nanoparticles acted as switches of T_2 measurement between aggregated and dispersed states, while with and without target bacteria. This MRS sensor can sensitively detect foodborne *P. aeruginosa* in the real food and drinking water samples with a detection limit of 50 CFU/mL [47].

The above protocols are all single-mode detection based on magnetic, so some scholars try to develop a dual-mode detection scheme. A protocol is proposed by Tyler et al. through the unique combination of magnetic and fluorescent parameters in a nanoparticle-based platform to construct a simple *Enterohemorrhagic Escherichia coli* O157:H7 diagnostic technique. This nano sensor was uniquely pair together magnetic relaxation and fluorescent modalities, allowing for a dual-detection platform. In the case of bacterial contamination, the binding between the magnetic nanoparticles and bacteria influence the transfer of surrounding water protons which causes a change in the T_2 relaxation times. As the concentration of bacteria in solution rises, the magnetic nanoparticles disperse and resulting in lower T_2 values. Conversely, fluorescence emission will increase in proportion with the concentration of bacteria, due to the increased number of magnetic nanoparticles directly bound to pathogen. This dual mode scheme can detect contamination with as low as 1 CFU present in solution within less than 1 h. Furthermore, the potential ability of them to be used in commercial packaged foods such as milk has been proved [48]. Subsequently, this group based on the similar dual-mode detection scheme to realize the detection of *Staphylococcus epidermidis* and *E. coli* which were contaminants in blood. This dual-mode determination improves the accuracy of actual detection [49].

However, the disadvantage of the MRS sensors depending on the state of magnetic particles is that the magnetic signal only positively correlated with the concentration of the target within a certain range, hence the linear range is narrow. And the state change is also susceptible to interference fcaused by various factors such as the sample matrix, which is easily suffered from the nonspecific adsorption and aggregation of magnetic particles that cause the inaccuracy of detection.

3.2 Amount-dependent MRS sensors for pathogens detection

The amount-dependent MRS sensors has proposed to solve the limitations of state-dependent MRS sensors. The basic scheme of MRS sensors based on the change of magnetic particles amounts depended on the difference in the separation speed of magnetic particles of different sizes in the same magnetic field. The magnetic particles of large diameter are used as the carrier of immunomagnetic separation, and the magnetic particles of small diameter are used as the magnetic signal probe. The donor/receptor specific recognition function molecular is modified on the both carrier and probe magnetic beads. The probe specifically recognizes the magnetic particles modified with the acceptor/donor through the carrier modified with the donor/receptor, and changes the number of magnetic probes after magnetic separation and other operations, thereby realizing biosensing. When the target appears and is recognized, the amount of magnetic probes is changed after magnetic separation, thereby realizing quantitative biosensing. This mode does not need to induce the aggregation of magnetic particles, which effectively improves the stability of MRS sensors. In addition, the T_2 signal is more sensitive to the change of magnetic probe concentration, which effectively improves the sensitivity of MRS sensors.

Chen et al. firstly proposed amount-dependent MRS sensor with more convenient operation, enhanced sensitivity and better reproducibility. Magnetic beads of large size (250 nm, MB250) can be separated more quickly than those of small size (30 nm, MB30) under an external magnetic field. Based on this phenomenon, a MRS sensor combined with magnetic separation that enables one-step, sensitive detection of pathogens. The MB250 and MB30 can selectively capture and enrich the targets to form the "MB250-target-MB30" conjugate. After magnetic separation, unreacted MB30 can be used as signal readout probe and corresponds to the concentration of targets (**Figure 4a**). The entire immunoassay can be completed within 30 min and the detection limit is 10^2 CFU/mL. Compared with conventional MRS sensor, this kind of sensors could avoid the unstable state of aggregation and ensure the accuracy of the signal, which is capable for the detection of *Salmonella* in milk [2]. Based on the similar principles, then this group proposed a highly sensitive magnetic DNA sensor based on nucleic acid hybridization reaction and magnetic signal readout. The scheme is to design the *L. monocytogenes* specific probe 1 and probe 2, and label them on the 30 and 250 nm magnetic nanoparticles, respectively. After hybridization reaction to form a sandwich nanocomplex and magnetic separation, the unbound 30 nm magnetic particles can act as the T_2 signal readout probe (**Figure 4b**). This assay allows the one-step detection of *L. monocytogenes* as low as 50 CFU/mL within 2 h without DNA amplification, providing a promising detection platform for pathogenic nucleic acid [50].

To integrate the amount-dependent technology and realize operate on 96-well plates, Zou et al. described a novel MRS sensor for *Salmonella* detection. In this

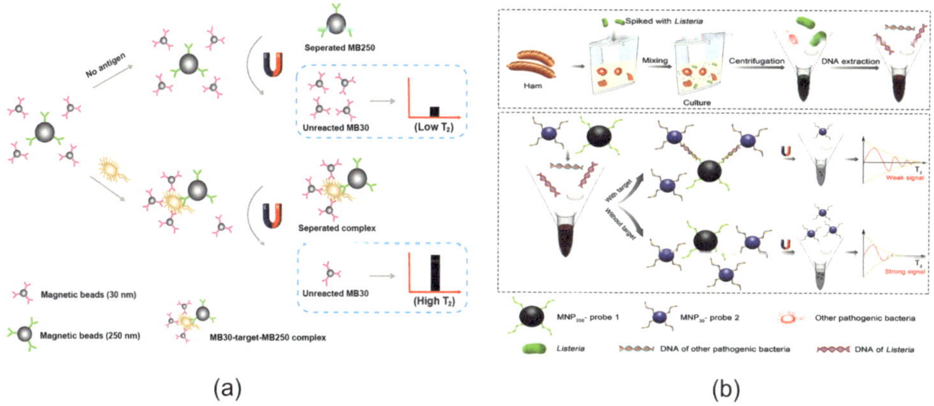

Figure 4.
(a) A MRS sensor based on the amounts of antibody-modified MNP for Salmonella *detection [2]; copyright 2015 American Chemical Society. (b) A MRS sensor based on the amounts of DNA-modified MNP for* L. monocytogenes *detection [50]. Copyright 2021 Elsevier.*

assay, functionalized Fe_3O_4 nanoparticle clusters (Fe_3O_4 NPC-SA) were used as probe to capture biotinylated antibody. The nanoparticles are cross-linked interaction and biotinylated antibody specifically recognize *Salmonella* at different sites. Then the Fe_3O_4 NPC-SA was eluted from 96-well microplates, which led to the change of transverse T_2. The strategy not only detected *Salmonella* at 10^5 CFU/mL showing high sensitivity, but also addressed a common phenomenon high-dose "hook effect" in which high concentration of analyte saturation prevents the effective aggregation of nanoparticles [51]. Similarly, Ling et al. combined membrane filtration with MRS sensor to establish a new time domain nuclear magnetic resonance (TD-NMR) biosensor to monitor and control *Salmonella* in milk for ensuring food safety, which also can overcomes the "hook effect" in MRS sensor. And the detection limits of pure culture solution and pasteurized milk were 2.3×10^3 CFU/mL [52]. Ting et al. developed dendritic superparamagnetic iron oxide nanoparticles(dendritic-SPIONs) combined with MRS sensor for *Salmonella* detection in milk. Bacterial capture antibody and biotinylated detection antibody (BT-mAb) were firstly used in the form of a sandwich in a 96-well plate to immobilize target pathogen. Then streptavidin modified polyamidoamine (SA-PAMAM) was used to connect BT-mAb and functionally modified SPIONs. PAMAM-mediated amplified functionalized SPIONs *via* streptavidin-biotin amplification system, aggregated nanoparticles to form dendritic SPIONs to achieve dual signal amplification. Finally, the dendritic SPIONs capture complex is eluted to test T_2 signal as the output of the target bacteria capture signal. This biosensor has detection limit of *Salmonella* in milk of 2.6×10^{4} CFU/mL, and showed good specificity to anti interference. Therefore, this innovative detection platform provides a novel signal amplification method [53]. These amount-dependent MRS sensors mentioned above can greatly expand the detection linear range, and avoid the interference from the sample matrix, which have the advantage of being more sensitive and stable. However, these methods still require the use of magnetic particles to convert the target signal into a relaxation signal.

3.3 Paramagnetic-ion mediated MRS sensors for pathogens detection

Conventional MRS assays employ monodispersed MNPs as the magnetic probe and modulate their states or amounts to result in the changes of transverse relaxation time of water protons. Nevertheless, the stability of MNPs when conjugating with the ligands remains an issue. The conjugation of MNPs may affect their stability, and the nonspecific interaction between MNPs and the sample matrix can result in the instability that affect the accuracy. The state-dependent and amount-dependent MRS sensors still need to be mediated by MNPs. The coupling procedure of the acceptor/donor on the surface of MNPs may be quite different for different operators, hence still insufficient for stability. Therefore, some researchers proposed novel paramagnetic ion-mediated MRS assays which have greatly improved the capability. It is much easier to prepare the aqueous solution of paramagnetic ions than that of MNPs. And its solution generally has a longer shelf life. Furthermore, paramagnetic ions have different valence states that can be interconverted by redox reactions, providing a versatile magnetic sensing platform. Wang et al. described a magnetic immunosensor relying on Mn(VII)/Mn(II) interconversion to trigger the corresponding change in the low-field nuclear magnetic resonance of the T_2. The signal of the water protons detected in Mn(II) aqueous solution is much stronger than Mn(VII) aqueous solution, hence enable to develop a background signal-free magnetic immunosensor with a high signal-to-background ratio through employ immunomagnetic separation and enzyme-catalyzed reaction (**Figure 5a**). The detection limit of this method for *Salmonella* is 20 CFU/mL, which has greatly improved the sensitivity of conventional paramagnetic ion-mediated magnetic sensors, offering a promising platform for bioanalysis [54]. On the basis of this mechanism, Li et al. presented an alkaline

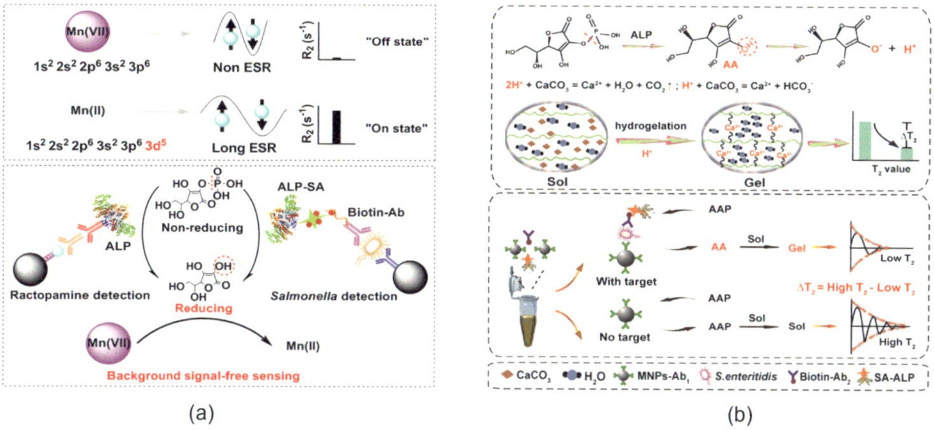

Figure 5.
(a) A paramagnetic ion Mn(VII)/Mn(II) mediated MRS sensor for Salmonella *detection [54]; copyright 2019 American Chemical Society. (b) A MRS sensor based on phosphatase-mediated transition of hydrogels for* Salmonella *detection [55]. Copyright 2021 American Chemical Society.*

Target	Limit of detection	Mode	References
Listeria monocytogenes	3 MPN	State-dependent	[41]
Cronobacter sakazakii	1.1 MPN	State-dependent	[42]
Salmonella	10^3 CFU/mL	State-dependent	[43]
Mycobacterium avium spp. *Paratuberculosis*	1.55 × 10^3 CFU/mL	State-dependent	[44]
Mycobacterium avium spp. *Paratuberculosis*	A single genome copy	State-dependent	[45]
Vibrio parahaemolyticus	10^5 CFU/mL	State-dependent	[46]
Pseudomonas aeruginosa	50 CFU/mL	State-dependent	[47]
Escherichia coli	1 CFU	State-dependent	[48]
Staphylococcus epidermidis and *E. coli*	2 CFU/mL	State-dependent	[49]
Salmonella	10^2 CFU/mL	Amount-dependent	[2]
Listeria monocytogenes	50 CFU/mL	Amount-dependent	[50]
Salmonella	10^5 CFU/mL	Amount-dependent	[51]
Salmonella	2.3 × 10^3 CFU/mL	Amount-dependent	[52]
Salmonella	2.6 × 10^4 CFU/mL	Amount-dependent	[53]
Salmonella	20 CFU/mL	Paramagnetic-ion	[54]
Listeria monocytogenes	10^2 CFU/mL	Paramagnetic-ion	[56]

Note: MPN—most probable number; CFU—colony forming unit.

Table 2.
Applications of MRS sensors in foodborne pathogens detection.

phosphatase (ALP)-mediated magnetic relaxation DNA biosensor enabling the rapid and sensitive analysis for *L. monocytogenes* in ham samples. The DNA probes were initially designed to specifically hybridize with targeted region of bacterial genomic DNA. And the amounts of ALP is related to the concentration of pathogen by DNA hybridization. Then ALP can induce Mn(VII) to convert into Mn(II) resulting in a significant change of T_2 signal through enzyme-catalyzed reaction. This MRS sensor could exhibit high sensitivity for *L. monocytogenes* detection with a low detection limit of 10^2 CFU/mL. The constructed simple and reliable DNA biosensor could offer an ideal candidate for the detection of foodborne pathogens [56].

In addition to catalyzing the redox of paramagnetic ion, the ALP can also participate in catalyzing the formation of hydrogels to cause the signal changes of T_2. Wei et al. developed a sol-gel transition of hydrogels to change T_2 signal for assaying foodborne pathogens. The ALP can catalyze the reaction to generate an acidic environment that could transform the sol-state alginate solution to hydrogel, and this process can directly regulate the diffusion rate of water protons resulting in the change of T_2 signal (**Figure 5b**). This biosensing strategy directly modulates the water molecules rather than conventional magnetic probes, hence displaying high sensitivity for detecting 50 CFU/mL *Salmonella* within 2 h and offering a straightforward and sensitive platform for pathogen detection [55]. The summary of different modes MRS sensors applied to foodborne pathogens detection are listed in **Table 2**.

4. Summary

This section mainly introduces the research progress of phage-based precise identification methods and magnetic relaxation switch sensors in the field of rapid detection for foodborne pathogens. Bacteriophage has strong specificity to pathogenic bacteria, easy to prepare, harmless to human body, can be used as a novel identification element to detect pathogenic bacteria. It mainly realized the rapid detection of foodborne pathogens by phage amplification, genetic engineering or detect the components. Besides, as a novel multidisciplinary analysis technology, the MRS sensors have the advantages of efficient analysis, high signal-to-noise ratio and simple operation, which is based on different scheme such as state, amounts and paramagnetic ion. The development of traditional MRS sensors are mature, but mainly relies on the state, mobility and distribution of hydrogen protons in the detection system, which have the disadvantage of insufficient sensitivity or targeting. Therefore, the targeting can be enhanced by developing novel functionalized nanoparticles while increasing sensitivity. With the deepening of research, the MRS sensors will play a more important role in the rapid detection of foodborne pathogens. The future research direction of MRS sensors can focus on multiple and high-throughput detection, achieve intelligent and portable on-site rapid detection, and exploring a revolutionary magnetic sensing mechanism. In the future, these emerging sensors based on specificity of phage and the efficient readout of MRS mentioned above will be developd rapidly for foodborne pathogens detection and contribute powerful methodological guarantee food safety, as well as human health.

Conflicts of interest

The authors declare that they have no known competing financial interests or personal relationships that could have appeared to influence the work reported in this paper.

Author details

Yiping Chen*, Junping Wen, Junpeng Zhao and Chenxi Huang
College of Food Science and Technology, Huazhong Agricultural University, Wuhan, Hubei, China

*Address all correspondence to: chenyiping@mail.hzau.edu.cn

IntechOpen

© 2022 The Author(s). Licensee IntechOpen. This chapter is distributed under the terms of the Creative Commons Attribution License (http://creativecommons.org/licenses/by/3.0), which permits unrestricted use, distribution, and reproduction in any medium, provided the original work is properly cited.

References

[1] Bayat F, Didar TF, Hosseinidoust Z. Emerging investigator series: Bacteriophages as nano engineering tools for quality monitoring and pathogen detection in water and wastewater. Environmental Science: Nano. 2021;**8**(2):367-389

[2] Chen Y, Xianyu Y, Wang Y, Zhang X, Cha R, Sun J, et al. One-step detection of pathogens and viruses: Combining magnetic relaxation switching and magnetic separation. ACS Nano. 2015;**9**(3):3184-3191

[3] Chen Y, Xianyu Y, Sun J, Niu Y, Wang Y, Jiang X. One-step detection of pathogens and cancer biomarkers by the naked eye based on aggregation of immunomagnetic beads. Nanoscale. 2016;**8**(2):1100-1107

[4] Shen Y, Xu L, Li Y. Biosensors for rapid detection of Salmonella in food: A review. Comprehensive Reviews in Food Science and Food Safty. 2021;**20**(1):149-197

[5] Chen C, Wang J. Optical biosensors: An exhaustive and comprehensive review. The Analyst. 2020;**145**(5):1605-1628

[6] García P, Martínez B, Obeso JM, Rodríguez A. Bacteriophages and their application in food safety. Letters in Applied Microbiology. 2008;**47**(6): 479-485

[7] Jamal M, Bukhari S, Andleeb S, Ali M, Raza S, Nawaz MA, et al. Bacteriophages: An overview of the control strategies against multiple bacterial infections in different fields. Journal of Basic Microbiology. 2019;**59**(2):123-133

[8] Farooq U, Yang Q, Ullah MW, Wang S. Bacterial biosensing: Recent advances in phage-based bioassays and biosensors. Biosensors and Bioelectronics. 2018;**118**:204-216

[9] Niyomdecha S, Limbut W, Numnuam A, Kanatharana P, Charlermroj R, Karoonuthaisiri N, et al. Phage-based capacitive biosensor for Salmonella detection. Talanta. 2018;**188**:658-664

[10] Rees CED, Dodd CER. Phage for rapid detection and control of bacterial pathogens in food. Advances in Applied Microbiology. 2006;**59**:159-186

[11] Rajnovic D, Muñoz-Berbel X, Mas J. Fast phage detection and quantification: An optical density-based approach. PLoS One. 2019;**14**(5):e0216292

[12] Garrido-Maestu A, Fuciños P, Azinheiro S, Carvalho C, Carvalho J, Prado M. Specific detection of viable Salmonella Enteritidis by phage amplification combined with qPCR (PAA-qPCR) in spiked chicken meat samples. Food Control. 2019;**99**:79-83

[13] Zhou Y, Marar A, Kner P, Ramasamy R. Charge-directed immobilization of bacteriophage on nanostructured electrode for whole-cell electrochemical biosensors. Analytical Chemistry. 2017;**89**(11):5734-5741

[14] Farooq U, Ullah MW, Yang Q, Aziz A, Xu J, Zhou L, et al. High-density phage particles immobilization in surface-modified bacterial cellulose for ultra-sensitive and selective electrochemical detection of Staphylococcus aureus. Biosensors and Bioelectronics. 2020;**157**:112163

[15] Tawil N, Sacher E, Mandeville R, Meunier M. Surface plasmon resonance

detection of *E. coli* and methicillin-resistant *S. aureus* using bacteriophages. Biosensors and Bioelectronics. 2012;**37**(1):24-29

[16] Singh A, Poshtiban S, Evoy S. Recent advances in bacteriophage based biosensors for food-borne pathogen detection. Sensors. 2013;**13**(2):1763-1786

[17] Chen J, Alcaine SD, Jiang Z, Rotello VM, Nugen SR. Detection of *Escherichia coli* in drinking water using T7 bacteriophage-conjugated magnetic probe. Analyrical Chemistry. 2015;**87**(17):8977-8984

[18] Peng Y, Jin Y, Lin H, Wang J, Khan MN. Application of the VPp1 bacteriophage combined with a coupled enzyme system in the rapid detection of Vibrio parahaemolyticus. Journal of Microbiological Methods. 2014;**98**:99-104

[19] Eed HR, Abdel-Kader NS, El Tahan MH, Dai T, Amin R. Bioluminescence-sensing assay for microbial growth recognition. Journal of Sensors. 2016;**2016**:1-5

[20] Klumpp J, Loessner MJ. Detection of bacteria with bioluminescent reporter bacteriophage. Bioluminescence: Fundamentals and Applications in Biotechnology. 2014;**144**:155-171

[21] van der Merwe RG, van Helden PD, Warren RM, Sampson SL, Gey van Pittius NC. Phage-based detection of bacterial pathogens. Analyst. 2014;**139**(11):2617-2626

[22] Smartt AE, Ripp S. Bacteriophage reporter technology for sensing and detecting microbial targets. Analytical Bioluminescence and Chemiluminescence. 2011;**400**(4): 991-1007

[23] Alcaine SD, Law K, Ho S, Kinchla AJ, Sela DA, Nugen SR. Bioengineering bacteriophages to enhance the sensitivity of phage amplification-based paper fluidic detection of bacteria. Biosensors and Bioelectronics. 2016;**82**:14-19

[24] Pande J, Magdalena S, Grover AK. Phage display: Concept, innovations, applications and future. Biotechnology Advances. 2010;**28**(6):849-858

[25] McIvor MJ, Karoonuthaisiri NT, Elliott C, Grant IR. Phage display-derived binders able to distinguish Listeria monocytogenes from other Listeria species. PLoS One. 2013;**8**(9):e74312

[26] Karoonuthaisiri N, Charlermroj R, Morton MJ, Oplatowska-Stachowiak M, Grant IR, Elliott CT. Development of a M13 bacteriophage-based SPR detection using Salmonella as a case study. Sensors and Actuators B: Chemical. 2014;**190**:214-220

[27] Golshahi L, Lynch KH, Dennis JJ, Finlay WH. In vitro lung delivery of bacteriophages KS4-M and PhiKZ using dry powder inhalers for treatment of Burkholderia cepacia complex and Pseudomonas aeruginosa infections in cystic fibrosis. Journal of Applied Microbiology. 2011;**110**(1):106-117

[28] Singh A, Arutyunov D, McDermott MT, Szymanskic CM, Evoy S. Specific detection of Campylobacter jejuni using the bacteriophage NCTC 12673 receptor binding protein as a probe. The Analyst. 2011;**136**(22):4780-4786

[29] Poshtiban S, Javed MA, Arutyunov D, Singh A, Banting G, Szymanski CM, et al. Phage receptor binding protein-based magnetic enrichment method as an aid for real time PCR detection of

foodborne bacteria. The Analyst. 2013;**138**(19):5619-5626

[30] Peng H, Chen IA. Rapid colorimetric detection of bacterial species through the capture of gold nanoparticles by chimeric phages. ACS Nano. 2019;**13**:1244-1252

[31] Tolba M, Ahmed MU, Tlili C, Eichenseher F, Loessnerb MJ, Zourob M. A bacteriophage endolysin-based electrochemical impedance biosensor for the rapid detection of Listeria cells. The Analyst. 2012;**137**(24):5749-5756

[32] Chibli H, Ghali H, Park S, Peterb Y-A, Nadeau JL. Immobilized phage proteins for specific detection of staphylococci. The Analyst. 2014;**139**(1):179-186

[33] Brzozowska E, Śmietana M, Koba M, Górska S, Pawlik K, Gamian A, et al. Recognition of bacterial lipopolysaccharide using bacteriophage-adhesin-coated long-period gratings. Biosensors and Bioelectronics. 2015;**67**:93-99

[34] Jun Y-W, Lee J-H, Cheon J. Chemical design of nanoparticle probes for high-performance magnetic resonance imaging. Angewandte Chemie (International Ed. in English). 2008;**47**(28):5122-5135

[35] Perez JM, Josephson L, O'Loughlin T, Hogemann D, Weissleder R. Magnetic relaxation switches capable of sensing molecular interactions. Nature Biotechnology. 2002;**20**(8):816-820

[36] Akbarzadeh A, Samiei M, Davaran S. Magnetic nanoparticles: Preparation, physical properties, and applications in biomedicine. Nanoscale Research Letters. 2012;**7**(144):1-13

[37] Shapiro MG, Westmeyer GG, Romero PA, Szablowski JO, Küster B, Shah A, et al. Directed evolution of a magnetic resonance imaging contrast agent for noninvasive imaging of dopamine. Nature Biotechnology. 2010;**28**(3):264-270

[38] Shao H, Min C, Issadore D, Liong M, Yoon T-J, Weissleder R, et al. Magnetic nanoparticles and microNMR for dagnostic applications. Theranostics. 2012;**2**(1):55-65

[39] Min C, Shao H, Liong M, Yoon T-J, Weissleder R, Lee H. Mechanism of magnetic relaxation switching sensing. ACS Nano. 2012;**6**(8):6821-6828

[40] Zhang Y, Yang H, Zhou Z, Huang K, Yang S, Han G. Recent advances on magnetic relaxation switching assay-based nanosensors. Bioconjugate Chemistry. 2017;**28**(4):869-879

[41] Zhao Y, Li Y, Jiang K, Wang J, White WL, Yang S, et al. Rapid detection of Listeria monocytogenes in food by biofunctionalized magnetic nanoparticle based on nuclear magnetic resonance. Food Control. 2017;**71**:110-116

[42] Zhao Y, Yao Y, Xiao M, Chen Y, Lee CCC, Zhang L, et al. Rapid detection of Cronobacter sakazakii in dairy food by biofunctionalized magnetic nanoparticle based on nuclear magnetic resonance. Food Control. 2013;**34**(2):436-443

[43] Wang S, Zhang Y, An W, Wei Y, Liu N, Chen Y, et al. Magnetic relaxation switch immunosensor for the rapid detection of the foodborne pathogen Salmonella enterica in milk samples. Food Control. 2015;**55**:43-48

[44] Kaittanis C, Naser SA, Perez JM. One-step, nanoparticle-mediated bacterial detection with magnetic relaxation. Nano Letters. 2007;**7**(2):380-383

[45] Kaittanis C, Boukhriss H, Santra S, Naser SA, Perez JM. Rapid and

sensitive detection of an intracellular pathogen in human peripheral leukocytes with hybridizing magnetic relaxation nanosensors. PLoS One. 2012;**7**(4):e35326

[46] Hash S, Martinez-Viedma MP, Fung F, Han JE, Yang P, Wong C, et al. Nuclear magnetic resonance biosensor for rapid detection of Vibrio parahaemolyticus. Biomedical Journal. 2019;**42**(3):187-192

[47] Jia F, Xu L, Yan W, Wu W, Yu Q, Tian X, et al. A magnetic relaxation switch aptasensor for the rapid detection of Pseudomonas aeruginosa using superparamagnetic nanoparticles. Microchimica Acta. 2017;**184**(5):1539-1545

[48] Shelby T, Sulthana S, McAfee J, Banerjee T, Santra S. Foodborne pathogen screening using magneto-fluorescent nanosensor: Rapid detection of E. Coli O157:H7. Journal of Visualized Experiments. 2017;**127**:1-7

[49] Banerjee T, Tummala T, Elliott R, Jain V, Brantley W, Hadorn L, et al. Multimodal magneto-fluorescent nanosensor for rapid and specific detection of blood-borne pathogens. ACS Applied Nano Materials. 2019;**2**(9):5587-5593

[50] Qia X, Wang Z, Lu R, Liu J, Li Y, Chen Y. One-step and DNA amplification-free detection of Listeria monocytogenes in ham samples: Combining magnetic relaxation switching and DNA hybridization reaction. Food Chemistry. 2021;**338**:127837

[51] Zou D, Jin L, Wu B, Hu L, Chen X, Huang G, et al. Rapid detection of Salmonella in milk by biofunctionalised magnetic nanoparticle cluster sensor based on nuclear magnetic resonance. International Dairy Journal. 2019;**91**:82-88

[52] Jin L, Li T, Wu B, Yang T, Zou D, Liang X, et al. Rapid detection of Salmonella in milk by nuclear magnetic resonance based on membrane filtration superparamagnetic nanobiosensor. Food Control. 2020;**110**:107011

[53] Li T, Jin L, Feng K, Yang T, Yue X, Wu B, et al. A novel low-field NMR biosensor based on dendritic superparamagnetic iron oxide nanoparticles for the rapid detection of Salmonella in milk. Lwt. 2020;**133**:110149

[54] Wang Z, Xianyu Y, Zhang Z, Guo A, Li X, Dong Y, et al. Background signal-free magnetic bioassay for food-borne pathogen and residue of veterinary drug via Mn(VII)/Mn(II) interconversion. ACS Sensors. 2019;**4**(10):2771-2777

[55] Wei L, Wang Z, Feng C, Xianyu Y, Chen Y. Direct transverse relaxation time biosensing strategy for detecting foodborne pathogens through enzyme-mediated sol-gel transition of hydrogels. Analtical Chemistry. 2021;**93**(17):6613-6619

[56] Li Y, Wu L, Wang Z, Tu K, Pan L, Chen Y. A magnetic relaxation DNA biosensor for rapid detection of Listeria monocytogenes using phosphatase-mediated Mn(VII)/Mn(II) conversion. Food Control. 2021;**125**:107959